Your Body

Praise for *Your Body*

"*Your Body*'s . . . redefinition of health and disease allows readers a deeper glimpse and redefinition of mind/body processes that, in turn, imparts a greater understanding of the evolutionary growth of both . . . [It] is . . . a 'book supporting life' . . . highly recommended for students of health and wellness, physical and mental healing, philosophy, and spirituality."
— *Diane Donovan, Midwest Book Review* —

"Everything Christopher McKeon offers in *Your Body* was completely new to me as a reader. His writing is eloquent and it's clear that his research has been exhaustive. His understanding of the information he offers is a combination of experience and intensive practice, and he has a genuine interest in bettering the lives of his readers on all levels . . . [His] tone is reassuring and confident, and I particularly appreciate that he increases a reader's sense of agency over their own bodies that extends far beyond the physical. Very highly recommended."
— *Jamie Michele, Readers' Favorite* —

"Concepts are broken down into bite-sized chunks in a linear progression for easy digestion . . . This volume is more practical . . . [and] serves as a manual for healing oneself and others . . . The personal accounts are convincing . . . Healing is the book's goal. Many self-help guides of a similar vein start with what's wrong (pain). This book begins with the fact that readers are well. The book shows how to access the health and wholeness within reach. Its tenor is affirming and encouraging."
— *Mari Carlson, US Review of Books* —

Books by Christopher McKeon

HEALING THROUGH AWARENESS series
The Story of Life
The Big Healing

Other Books
Victim to Victor

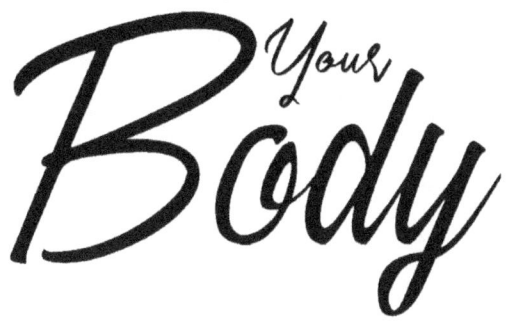

Your Body

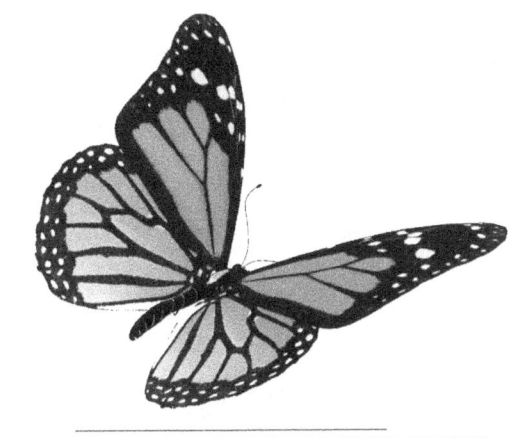

CHRISTOPHER MCKEON
M.DIV.

Rico

Tōteppit Press
2025

Tōteppit Press
Rico, Colorado USA

www.toteppitpress.com

Copyright © 2025 by Christopher McKeon.

All rights reserved under International, Pan-American, and other relevant Copyright Conventions. No part of this book may be changed, modified, edited, used, or reproduced in any manner or for money or any sort of remuneration whatsoever without written permission from the Publisher, except for brief quotations embodied in critical articles and reviews properly cited. Photocopying portions of this book is permissible within the scope of applicable copyright law and for private use. This book is personal revelatory testimony and does not constitute advice, medical or otherwise.

Publisher's Cataloging-in-Publication Data
McKeon, Christopher D.A., author.
Your body: a course in healing / Christopher McKeon.
Rico, CO: Tōteppit Press, 2025. | Series: Healing through awareness, bk. 3. | Includes bibliographical references and index. | Also available in audiobook format.
LCCN 2024924401 (print) | ISBN 979-8-9864707-9-5 (paperback) | ISBN 978-1-966345-00-8 (hardcover) | ISBN 978-1-966345-01-5 (ebook)
LCSH: Healing. | Mental healing. | Subconsciousness. | Alternative medicine. | Self-actualization. | Illustrated works. | BISAC: BODY, MIND & SPIRIT / Healing / General. | BODY, MIND & SPIRIT / Inspiration & Personal Growth. | HEALTH & FITNESS / Healing. | SELF-HELP / Personal Growth / General.
LCC RZ401 .M35 2025 (print) | LCC RZ401 (ebook) | DDC615.8/51–dc23.

Cover design by rebeccacovers
Cover image: "The Challenge" by Mark Rode Sculpture, Ireland, with permission
Chapter pages image: vecteezy.com with permission
Text set in EB Garamond

HAMLET
What / have you, my good friends, deserved at the hands of
Fortune that she sends you to prison hither?
GUILDENSTERN
Prison, my lord?
HAMLET
Denmark's a prison.
ROSENCRANTZ
Then is the world one.
HAMLET
A goodly one, in which there are many confines,
wards, and dungeons, Denmark being one o'
th' worst.
ROSENCRANTZ
We think not so, my lord.
HAMLET
Why, then, 'tis none to you, for *there is
nothing either good or bad but thinking makes it
so.* To me, it is a prison.
ROSENCRANTZ
Why, then, your ambition makes it one.
'Tis too narrow for your mind.
HAMLET
O God, I could be bounded in a nutshell and
count myself a king of infinite space . . .
—Shakespeare *Hamlet* 2.2.258–274 (emph. add.)

With gratitude for
my daughter Ayako
— & —
Cindy, Tony, and Simon

Contents

Page

Preface   *i*
What's in It for You   *v*

1. What Is Human Life?   1

Emergence	2
You as a Self-aware Proto-energy Being	2
Emergent Proto-energy	3
Way of Being	4
*L*ife Force	5
Self-awareness	5
Physical Embodiment	6
Physicospirit	9
Transcendence of *L*ife	10
The Corruption	12
The Negative Collective Consciousness	13
The Universe in Which You Live	15
How the Physical Environment Powers the Spirit One	18
Summary of Chapter 1	20

2. How Your Body Works in Our Universe   23

1 What Is the Body	25
1.1 All Existence	26
1.1.1 Emergence Defined	26
1.1.2 Energent-prime Intelligence	27
1.1.3 Way of Being	30
1.1.4 The Principal Aspects of All Existence	31
1.2 Your Mind	31
1.3 Embodiment	32
2 Origin of the Body	33
2.1 Rise of the Humans	34
2.1.1 Emergent Birth of the First Humans	35
2.1.1.1 Sex	37
2.1.1.2 Proto-love	39
2.1.2 The Meaning of *H*uman	40
2.2 Building the Human Body	42
2.2.1 Evolution of the Human Body	43
2.2.1.1 Directed and Undirected Evolution	43
2.2.2 Developing the Body's Form	44
2.2.3 The Body Takes Shape	45
2.2.4 The Spirit Body Experience	48
2.3 Birth of You and Your Body	49
2.3.1 Energent Proto-life	50
2.3.2 Emergent Birth of *L*ife	53
2.3.2.1 Birth of *L*ife: Phase One	54
2.3.2.2 Birth of *L*ife: Phase Two	54
2.3.2.3 Birth of *L*ife: Phase Three	55
2.3.3 Birth of Your Physicospirit Body	55
2.3.4 Conclusion to Origin of the Body	56
3 The Milieu in Which Your Body Lives	57
3.1 Space Infinity	57
3.2 Fundamental Energent	59
3.2.1 The Energent of Our Universe	60

      3.2.2 'On-Off' Proto-energy — 62
      3.2.3 You as Emergent 𝓛ife — 64
      3.2.4 Conclusion to Fundamental Energent — 65
   3.3 Physical Universe Energies — 65
      3.3.1 Energy — 65
      3.3.2 Matter (of Which Your Body Is Made) — 66
         3.3.2.1 Archí — 66
      3.3.3 Existent 'Energy' — 67
         3.3.3.1 Enérgeia — 68
   3.4 Conclusion to the Milieu in Which Your Body Lives — 69
4 Mind and Body — 69
   4.1 Nonhuman Mind-Brain-Body — 70
      4.1.1 Instantiation of Nonhuman Mind — 70
      4.1.2 Nonhuman Brain-body Integration — 72
   4.2 Human Mind-Brain-Body — 72
      4.2.1 Physical Mind as Facsimile of 𝓛ife Mind — 72
   4.3 Mind-body Integration — 76
      4.3.1 Self-awareness — 76
      4.3.2 Human Mind-body Integration — 77
5 Infinity of Psyche — 79
   5.1 Event Periodicity — 81
   5.2 Consciousness and Reality — 81
   5.3 Omniscience, Omnipresence, Omnipotence, Omniexistence — 83
6 Way of Being — 86
   6.1 All Existence Way of Being — 86
   6.2 Self-organized Way of Being — 87
   6.3 𝕳uman Way of Being — 88
      6.3.1 Accountableism, Culture, and Ultraculture — 88
      6.3.2 Way of Being of the Physical Body — 89
      6.3.3 Emergent Way of Being — 90
      6.3.4 Emergence of 𝓛ife — 90
7 Conclusion to Chapter 2 — 91

3. The Bell of the Mind   95

1 The Nature of Mind — 95
2 Experience of Mind — 98
   2.1 Subconscious-conscious Mind — 98
      2.1.1 Subconscious and Mind-body Integration — 101
      2.1.2 What is Subconscious 'Belief' — 102
         2.1.2.1 Why Subconscious Experiences 'Energy' as It Does — 103
         2.1.2.2 Why Corruption 'Energy' Is Subconscious 'Energy' — 107
   2.2 Conscious Awareness of Subconscious — 109
      2.2.1 Subconscious Intentionality Exerts on Conscious Mind — 110
3 Intentionality — 112
4 The Bell of the Mind — 112
   4.1 The Way of 'Energy' — 113
   4.2 How Your Subconscious Experiences 'Energy' — 115
5 Conclusion to Chapter 3 — 117

4. How the Body Malfunctions   119

1 Damage/Injury — 121
   1.1 Damage — 121
   1.2 Injury — 122
   1.3 Why Disease — 122

		1.3.1 Emotive Expression: Emotive *L*ife Force	123
	1.4	Why Aging?	125
	1.5	Why Death?	126

5. What Is a Malfunction 129
1. Intentionality From Own-self Mind — 131
2. Intentionality From Other-self Mind — 133
   - 2.1 Ultraculture — 134

6. Intentionality 137
1. Awareness — 139
2. Psyche Fundamental Force — 140
   - 2.1 How PFF Works — 141
     - 2.1.1 God Speaking Creation Into Existence — 143
3. Natural (Physical-world) Intentionality — 143
   - 3.1 How Intentionality Works — 144
   - 3.2 Step 1: Formulate Desire as Force of Thought — 145
     - 3.2.1 Consider What You Want to Accomplish — 145
     - 3.2.2 Formulate Way of Being — 146
     - 3.2.3 Invest Thought with Reality — 146
   - 3.3 Step 2: Exert Force of Thought into the Environment — 148
     - 3.3.1 Focus *L*ife Force — 149
     - 3.3.2 Exert the Focus — 150
   - 3.4 Physical-self Intentionality — 150
4. How to Exert Intentional Energy — 151
   - 4.1 Your Physically Instantiated 'Subconscious' — 154
   - 4.2 Exerting Intentional Energy — 156
     - 4.2.1 The Exertion — 157
   - 4.3 Intentional Focus, Force, Strength, and Power — 159
     - 4.3.1 Focus — 159
     - 4.3.2 Force — 160
     - 4.3.3 Strength — 160
     - 4.3.4 Power — 160

7. Transforming Regular Damage 161
1. Understanding Emergent Way of Being — 161
   - 1.1 Your Body's Dual Way of Being — 163
     - 1.1.1 Attributive Way of Being — 164
2. How Subconscious Swaps Emergent for Attributive WoB — 167
3. How to Manifest Emergent WoB and Avoid Chronic Damage — 168

8. Transforming Damage from Your Own Mind 169
1. Intentionally Heal the Damage — 169
   - 1.1 What is a Trained Healer? — 170
2. Damage Can't Exist If You Don't Want It — 172
   - 2.1 Permanent Healing — 172
3. Psyche Healing — 173
   - 3.1 What Is Healing — 173
     - 3.1.1 Healing and Harm — 174
     - 3.1.2 Healing Is Neutralizing Negative Em*L*f — 175
     - 3.1.3 Prerequisite to Healing — 176
     - 3.1.4 Healing Oneself — 177
   - 3.2 How Psyche Healing Works — 177
     - 3.2.1 Healing by Letting Go Pain and Suffering — 178
     - 3.2.2 Neutralizing Negative Em*L*f — 178
     - 3.2.3 Healing by Mina — 179

	3.2.3.1 Step 1: Encompassing the Individual with Mina's *Life* force		180
	3.2.3.2 Step 2: An Awareness That One's Pain Never Happened		181
	3.2.3.3 Step 3: Resetting Awareness of 'Energy' of Human Way of Being		181
4	Conclusion to Chapters 7 and 8		183
	4.1 My 'Dumpster Fire' Healing		184

9. Transforming Damage from Others' Intentionality   185

1. Awareness of an Attack — 189
   1.1 Intentional Attack — 189
2. Neutralize an Attack's Energy — 190
3. Conclusion to Chapters 1–9 — 191
   3.1 Energy Testing — 192
      3.1.1 What Is Chakra Energy — 192
      3.1.2 Chakra Health — 193
      3.1.3 The Aura — 194

10. Testimonies   195

1. Simon — 195
2. Shelley — 200
3. Scott — 203
4. Tony — 204
5. Harriet — 206
6. Amelia — 209

Endnotes   217
Works Cited   219
Index   221

Preface

Your Body is a follow up and companion work to *The Story of Life* (SOL; McKeon 2022), which I wrote over a four-year period to introduce our true human existence and Mina, whom most would liken to God. He's the human person who built our universe with its physical and spirit environments along with our physical body although not *you*, the *person*.

This book is also the culmination of seven years working with Mina to learn about humanity's spirit reality as well as psyche (mind) and physical body healing. This book relies on *energy testing* to converse with Mina and other spirit persons. Energy testing substitutes for our spirit senses because our current level of mind–brain integration doesn't support them in the way we typically imagine spirit mediums communicating with the so-called dead, angels, or God.

Unlike with spirit mediums, the beauty of energy testing is that you can learn it and validate for yourself what you read in this book and *The Story of Life* similar to how scientists validate other scientists' experiments and conclusions in their own labs. In this respect, energy testing is a scientific method. I encourage you to join the global energy testing community (toteppitpress.com/et-community).

The Story of Life extensively teaches about our physical body in the context of its integration with our spirit embodiment and overarching mind. Yet, it really only summarizes physical embodiment because there's just a lot to take in despite its gargantuan 700 pages. *The Big Healing* (TBH; McKeon 2024) is *The Story of Life*'s action-packed first 10 chapters in a larger font with only 236 pages. It follows my daughters' and my discovery of, and initial experience with, Mina. You may find it a more easily digestible introduction to *The Story of Life*.

Mina asked me to write this book to provide a more detailed understanding of how your physical body works in the context of our universe and psyche (mind) healing; why your body *malfunctions* into illness, disease, chronic pain or injury, aging, and death; what a malfunction actually is;

and how the body *transforms* from that condition to its original, *emergent Way of Being* (what most folks think of as perfect health and wellbeing).

Bear in mind this book provides only an overview of fundamental concepts that are absolutely essential such as All Existence, proto-energy, the Energent, and ℒife that *The Story of ℒife* elucidates in detail. They aren't necessary for a healer to heal your body, but are essential for you to master self-healing. Cross-references to *The Story of ℒife* are written as SOL §#:*page#* that point to further, useful reading. In a citation, *io* and *ia* mean italics original or italics added. To keep this book a reasonable length, I cross-reference *The Story of ℒife* extensively although key concepts get brief explanations here. Cross-references to sections within this book are written as chapter#§#:*page#* sometimes with CHAPTER-NAME for clarity.

Chapter 2 and parts of Chapters 1 and 6 cover the basic, necessary information you need to comprehend energy and 'energy' toward understanding the physical matter of your body as manifested 'energy.' When in single quotes, 'energy' is referencing a different aspect of energy having nothing to do with kinetic or potential physical energies like electromagnetism or stored energies that you're maybe used to. Chapter 2 is the longest by far. It's an essential primer to understand your body in the milieu, or context, in which it lives. It helps you understand why your mind can heal it instead of only doctors, God, wishful thinking, hope, faith, or whatever you use to live one day to the next without falling ill, maimed, into pain, or unexpectedly dead.

Chapters 3–5 cover your subconscious–conscious mind, how your body malfunctions, and what a malfunction is. Chapter 6 teaches you how to Intentionalize your thought. Chapters 7–9 describe healing the malfunctions of your body. Chapter 10 presents testimonies by individuals who've experienced healing as this book describes.

I've striven to provide the critical details you need to experience physical healing, but the concepts herein can only be truly comprehended by thoughtfully reading *The Story of ℒife*. The print version is the best way to take in the book but the Kindle and PDF are free (toteppitpress.com/downloadsolpdf) and we offer free paperbacks when SOL book sales provide sufficient funding. Or consider a 5-day seminar (chrismckeon.com/events). The text explains all terms unique to this book. An index gives you a handy quick reference.

The fundamental purpose of *The Story of ℒife* and this book is *healing through awareness*. This means that, in gaining an understanding of your physical and spirit reality, your mindset naturally transforms (consciously or subconsciously, depending on you) and leads to healing your psyche's pain and suffering and, accordingly, your body. Don't give up if the concepts seem too out of the box or difficult. Let your subconscious absorb it even though your conscious mind may not. Keep in mind this is not a medical book. It is not promising healing but teaching how it's possible to achieve it. Healing is different for each person because he or she consciously or subconsciously chooses what they want.

As one of my students said, "I sit down every day, absorbing the content with a new vision of myself and the universe that the author is revealing in his compelling book.

"I read it again and again to capture its depth and breadth. Like snorkeling or deep sea diving, there is always something new to discover in becoming aware of how I can make a difference in my life and in the world, too.

"The writing pops out at me through an amazing awareness I didn't have during previous reads. I feel my environment changing as I gain dominion over every event in my life. I am daily healing my body from accidents and illness.

"At first, the magnitude of the information was difficult to wrap my head around. But I take to heart what the author penned: to not let it overwhelm me, to let my subconscious absorb it as I read. It continues to be an amazing journey of one revelation upon another. The more I read the more it makes sense. This is the best resource for healing that I've ever encountered. It gives such a rich blend of detail of the completeness of our world and of practical applications that help build my awareness necessary for healing and ultimate health and wellbeing . . . my journey continues daily."

I hope this book brings such real healing to you . . . because life is all about happiness, not suffering.

Christopher Mckeon
Southwest Colorado, USA
January 2025

What's in It for You

More than once upon a time I injured myself. Doctors filled me with hope I could walk it off. That it was short-term. Fixable. Then I couldn't and it wasn't.

They said, "Oops! Looks incurable. A chronic condition. So sorry!"

I said, "Meh!" and trained myself to grin and bear the pain, debility, and depression. My new life of suffering.

Maybe I deserved it. Was it punishment? karma? my special spiritual growth path from the God of Love or the faceless bureaucrats of reincarnation? Regardless, I longed for a way out that didn't involve dying. Then, in 2017, I discovered I could heal and heal I did!

How about you? Does your body feel like a rusty jalopy on its way to the scrapyard? Are you longing for relief? You deserve to heal—*transform*—your body not to mention your psyche (consciousness; mind). The awesome news is that, with awareness of your human reality, you can! In this book, you'll learn why and how illness, disease, chronic injury, even aging happens and can be reversed and removed without a coincidental bank transfusion to the Lofty Promise industry ever swilling new life from yours like a Transylvanian Count.

Mina, the human person whom humanity thinks of as God or a god who created—built—our universe and our physical bodies, did not create *us*. We are, each of us, *emergently birthed beings*. If you think your body, other people, the natural world, God, or whatever you can imagine controls you . . . well, I invite you to think again. Whatever it is that you experience, you have consciously or subconsciously enabled and accepted for reasons of your own. *Ouch.*

That was a hard pill to swallow when two of my daughters and I met Mina. But gravel it down we did, because he made the case. It brought me a sense of liberation, peace, and happiness I'd have scoffed at only one day earlier.

"You're not your body," Mina said. "You emergently birth as 'energy.'"

"Aren't I just mind? Or maybe brain?" The gods of science had certainly hammered that notion home.

My third daughter El was energy testing for the three of us. She chuckled. "He's laughing, Dad. He says our mind transcends our physical embodiment, not to mention our spirit self."

"Isn't spirit supposed to be our ultimate existence?"

"He says no. And that you should know that after all your religious and spiritual experience."

"Ha ha. You sure that isn't you just—"

"I tested that's what he said. Ask Ayako to test if you don't trust me."

I swung eyes my oldest daughter Ayako's way but her palms pushed flat out. "She's right even without me checking her testing, Dad. I've known that a long time."

"How would you know that?"

"You don't want to know."

I burped a breath. "I sure do!" She scrunched a face through heavenward eyes.

Mina said through El, "Your mind, as 'energy,' is absolutely autonomous. It can't be invaded by any other mind. Whatever you do or experience, in some way it was your choice to make it happen."

"Pfft! Come on. I don't choose to get a cold. Or cancer. Or age. Who would even—"

"He means it's your subconscious mostly doing it," Ayako said. "It's experiencing and reacting to energies with Intentionality."

"Intentionality?" I popped what Ayako said to Mina myself. My body swayed *yes* like sludge. In these early days closing out 2017, the girls were lightyears ahead of me when it came to the 'energy' sensitivity that's necessary to sway (energy) test with alacrity. But that was then. Now it's seven years later.

This was just a tidbit of what we learned (in different terms) that first night in our quaint log cabin in Virginia's heavy rural woods. The bottom line is that your emergently birthed self—what most think of as mind or beingness—*integrates* your body somewhat analogous to the driver of a car having some sort of brain interface. While your body has its own physical reality amongst the physical 'laws' of our physical universe, the fact it integrates your mind means that, despite its physical reality, it is fundamentally an extension of your mind just like your spirit body. Check out *The Big Healing* (*TBH*) for the full monty with my daughters or else *The Story of Life* for the big picture. In the seven years since that shocking

Virginia night, Mina taught me everything you'll read in this book never mind the whole shooting match that's *The Story of Life*. You won't find anything on Earth like it nor anyone else who knows it.

If you're struggling with illness, disease, chronic pain, or injury then what you learn in this book can free you from the yoke of false beliefs that literally prevents your body from healing itself in accord with *emergent Way of Being*. The healing you're about to discover has demonstrable results. We showcase some of these in Chapter 10's testimonies. Each chapter provides new secrets that will help you control your physical body as well as your life here on Earth. If you accept the information this book reveals and give your mind the chance to let go its old, harmful beliefs, it's highly possible you can enjoy the rest of your physical life unburdened by bodily pain and suffering. Don't delay! You might not get a second chance. Turn the page and let's get you started on the path to healing and health *right now*!

What Is Human Life?

This chapter is a brief overview of the book. We get into the real nitty gritty of healing your physical body beginning with Chapter 2. All the terms and concepts in this chapter are defined and described throughout the book and can be found in the index.

Before describing how your body works and why it suffers illness, chronic injury, and death, and before you can successfully heal your body, you need awareness that you are a *physicospirit* person—the physically alive individual plus spirit (embodied) self—and that life itself transcends physical existence. This means your physical human body is an *embodiment* and not, in and of itself, a *being*. What *is* a being, however, is what *The Story of Life* calls ℒife (McKeon 2022, § 1.2:246). ℒife is *you*: an *emergently birthed self-aware proto-energy person*, not an artifact of physical conception nor a biological entity.

No human, divine, or any other being has the creational power to 'make' a ℘erson, where ℘erson means the totality that is mind where mind is ℘erson and ℘erson is ℒife. A physical human person is merely the ℘erson integrating an evolved *proto-human body* having the Intentional, *pairwise* capability to 'trigger' emergent birth of ℒife 'in' *Energent proto-life* via sexual reproduction . . . don't worry, we'll explain all these terms. Three examples of proto-human are the anatomically correct 'humans' prior to about 50,000 years ago, Neanderthals, and you the zygote before dividing from two cells to four. Humans since about 50,000 years ago—you and me—are nobody's creations. Each of us uniquely *births* as *emergent* ℒife that integrates a physical body.

We describe the concept of *emergence* in CH. 2 § 1.1.1:26. For now, think of emergence as an entity that self-organizes into existence that is, even in principle, unpredictable and novel. Its properties are not inherent to its constituents nor can be inferred or predicted from them. An example is the wetness of water from two hydrogen atoms and one oxygen atom where wetness is more than the sum of the properties of its parts . . . it's an *emergent property*.

Emergence

"Emergence is a spontaneous, bottom-up, self-organizing phenomenon of complexity, with no external cause required, no top-down design and no centralized control of the system" (Lewis 2023). You, as an emergently birthed being, are an *emergence* of ℒife. Uncreated by any being. Not the result of any being. Emergently unique.

The Story of ℒife calls 'all there infinitely is' *All Existence*. All Existence comprises *proto-energy*; we call it this because it is the fundamental 'energy' of 'all there infinitely is' and it's unlike any energy that humanity has discovered or imagined. It is without space or time. We call the proto-energy of All Existence *Energent–prime*, as it's the root of the proto-energy that powers the existence of our universe. We call the proto-energy of our universe simply *Energent*.

You as a Self-aware Proto-energy Being

There is an emergent property of Energent–prime that we call *Energent proto-life*. It's a ℒife-precursor proto-energy without space or time. References to space and time in the context of Energent proto-life are written in single quotes as 'space,' 'time,' 'in,' 'out of,' and so forth. Energent proto-life is a ℒife-precursor because, when triggered, Energent proto-life emergently coalesces, differentiates, and self-organizes at a unique 'point in space' *as* ℒife, the human person.

In essence, the person is simply self-aware proto-energy having ℒife, where ℒife is the properties and characteristics that emergently birth 'in' Energent proto-life via pairwise sexual reproduction. Emergent self-aware proto-energy is the fundamental beingness of the person who is infinite, meaning indeterminate, in that the person isn't limited by time and space and instantly *is* wherever their awareness is. All Existence is indeterminate. It has this property because it is proto-energy's Way of Being. Energent proto-life, an emergent property of Energent–prime, is accordingly indeterminate, too.

*L*ife—*you*—which is an emergent property of Energent proto-life that's triggered by pairwise humans *is* an emergently self-aware All Existence. In consequence, *L*ife inherits properties—proto-energy; existence, time, and spatial indeterminateness; emergent Way of Being—that give rise to such heretofore deific attributes as omnipotence, omnipresence, omniscience, and omniexistence. Emergent *L*ife—mind, thus ℘erson—is its own *absolutely autonomous* proto-energy self-existence (*SOL* § 1.2:563). This is why you, a human being who integrates a physical body, are an eternal being in both an indeterminate—infinite—environment *having no* space or time (All Existence) and an indeterminate environment *having* space and time (our universe).

The human person is a being of self-aware proto-energy, not a body. You are, in your essence, like a self-contained bubble of proto-energy. Because you emergently birth 'in' Energent proto-life, we call the self-aware proto-energy that is your fundamental beingness *emergent proto-energy*. Physical or spirit embodiment is merely how you interact as a discrete 'energy' being with what's external to your proto-energy self, such as our universe. You achieve this interaction using your mind, which is an aspect of your (self-aware) proto-energy self. You can't experience what's beyond your self-containment without mind. Think of mind as an interface between your proto-energy self and what's 'outside of,' or external to, it.

Emergent Proto-energy

Your spirit body, for example, is made of *supramatter*. This is matter in the context of the supranatural (spirit) environment of our universe. Supramatter's Way of Being is whatever human beings give it because it's entirely malleable by your mind. Accordingly, your mind *subconsciously* manifests your spirit body however it sees you. But you can *consciously* manifest your spirit body as any sex, age, height, size . . . whatever and however you like.

Your physical body, on the other hand, is made of matter. This is what science calls the physical stuff of our natural (physical) environment, our universe. Matter's Way of Being exists whether or not human persons interact with it. It's determined by the builder of a universe. But humans can alter matter's Way of Being using *Intentionality*. This is the exertion of 'mind energy' that affects the Energent proto-energy suffusing our universe, which in turn affects every scintilla of matter in it (CH. 6:137). This means that you can alter your physical body however your mind sees your embodied self. However, physical matter is more tedious to alter because its naturally independent Way of Being resists change, unlike supramatter's human-Intentionalized Way of Being which doesn't resist change. This is why physical healing takes time. Even so-called instant healing takes time from Mina's perspective. It's anywhere from a picosecond—a trillionth of a second—to twelve hours when a healer achieves that capability.

The key thing to comprehend about *emergent proto-energy* is that it's the 'energy' of which you are a being. It's as fundamental as it gets for you. When we refer to the human person as self-aware proto-energy, we're talking about the person in their *personness*. Emergent proto-energy references the person simply as the 'energy' of which one emergently births. Science references the person simply as the matter of the body, which is the energy of fundamental atomic forces and chemistry. Importantly for healing the physical body, however, emergent proto-energy even more fundamentally suffuses your physical embodiment. In effect, your physical body, despite being matter, is quite literally your emergent proto-energy. It *is* the 'energy' of your very beingness. This is the 'energy' that you affect via Intentionality to alter the physical matter of your body to transform, or heal, your physical health and wellbeing.

All Existence *is* Way of Being. Everything in the natural environment, too, *is* Way of Being. A cup, for instance, doesn't have or embody or

Way of Being   exert Way of Being. It simply *is* Way of Being, and that Way of Being is the fullness of the matter that we call a cup. You, yourself, *have* Way of Being. The reason we *have* it instead of *are* it is because we are absolutely autonomous, emergently birthed beings. Our autonomy arises in the Way of Being of our emergent birth. We have no fixed Way of Being like a cup except in terms of what we are as a self-aware proto-energy being. We can't remake ourselves into some other form of existence. We *are* emergent proto-energy having emergent Way of Being that *is* a self-aware proto-energy being. This is *Life*.

Our Way of Being is Human Way of Being, where Human is humanity in every collective sense as *Life* (SOL § 3:280). Human Way of Being is what makes us uniquely what's called *human*. It's what *The Story of Life* terms *emergent* Way of Being, which is the Way of Being of our emergent birth. Emergent Way of Being *is* the Way of Being of our physical body. It's what people think of as perfect health and eternal physical life.

Emergent Way of Being suffuses our emergent proto-energy, the latter incorporating the former while one and the same though not equivalent. Emergent Way of Being isn't a force or power or energy or any such thing. It is *Way of Being*; that's the only way to describe it. As emergent Way of Being suffuses emergent proto-energy and emergent proto-energy suffuses our physical body, emergent Way of Being suffuses the 'energy' of the matter–Energy of our body (note that *matter–Energy* is a more accurate understanding of matter and energy in relationship than Einstein's $E=mc^2$; SOL § 2:114). This suffused 'energy' is what people generally think of as the body's life force. *The Story of Life* calls it Life force.

Life force *is* our emergent proto-energy suffused with emergent Way of Being; not just emergent proto-energy on its own, but altogether. These are emergent properties of the Human person, not Intentionalized by another person but emergently birthing as novel Life. Life force is unique to the person regardless humanity's overarching Human Way of Being that's an aspect of the individual.

Life Force

Without *attributive Way of Being*—the Way of Being that every individual creates for themselves in their absolute autonomy through which they experience as reality that which they believe is real—our body naturally suffuses emergent Way of Being and therefore Life force. Your physical body *is* the 'energy' of your emergent proto-energy suffusing emergent Way of Being. In other words, your body naturally exists in perfect, eternal health without any effort on your part. The rub is ditching that pesky attributive Way of Being that, as the 'energy' of your proto-energy self, tells your body it's an animal subject to damage, biological attack, and death.

Generally, self-awareness comes in two flavors: nonhuman and human, the reason being that brain, in and of itself, instantiates nonhuman mind whereas Life, in and of itself, *is* mind (SOL § 1.1:246). Overall, self-awareness is the subjective experiential awareness of *own-self's* subjective experience of objective reality. It diminishes in scope indirectly proportional to the increase in primitivity.

Self-awareness

Let's define own-self. Anything that's alive has an intense interest in own-self wellbeing experiencing the world. This doesn't mean one's *own* psychosomatic sense of wellbeing but however one determines *own-self* wellbeing. Own-self is almost infinitely definable. For some, it means *me*. For others it means *my family, my job, my community-nation-planet, my cause, my God, anything-in-some-way-me-related*—singly or in combination—even at the expense of *me* (SOL § 1:94). Outside of human behavior, we don't observe own-self operating beyond the *me* except in gradations with certain mammals like dogs, dolphins, whales, elephants, chimps, and the like (SOL § 2:275). We see own-self represented, for example, in what French philosopher Jean-Jacques Rousseau (d. 1778) called two principles prior to reason, ". . . one of which interests us deeply in our own Preservation and Welfare, and the other inspires us with a natural Aversion to see any other Being, but especially any Being like ourselves, suffer or perish," the latter being wishful thinking (Rousseau 1761, *lv*).

Human self-awareness is the subjective experiential awareness of being subjectively aware of one's subjective experience of objective reality. Not as *qualia*—these are instances of subjective, ineffable conscious experiences as distinct from any physical or computational process—or as own-self in the totality of experience of which both are aspects, but as the autonomous experience of own-self itself. Human self-awareness is *Life* and entirely a function of the emergent person. This means a person has experiential awareness of own-self as though not own-self, as if they were a separate, equally autonomous observer. It's why a person can exist as though an autonomous entity apart from own-self yet experience own-self's subjective and objective reality *as* own-self while *not* own-self; to 'clinically detach' from self to experience self.

Self-awareness in average terms is a very limited experience because few people really engage it. Only certain spirit persons have ever pushed it to its absolute apparent limit. Even then, they can only ever know they've reached *their* limit and not *its* limit (*SOL* § 3:331). Finally, don't think that nonhuman self-awareness isn't real or only a faux version of human self-awareness. They differ only in degree not in kind.

Being a self-aware proto-energy person, your physical self directly experiences All Existence, or 'all there infinitely is,' beyond—external to—mind (*SOL* CH. 18:227). We might think that what is outside mind (a universe, say) is tangible reality whereas what's inside is merely intangible Thought... here, *consciousness* means the totality of self-aware experience and *mind* the totality of Thought, which is thinking–feeling in the totality of consciousness (*SOL* § 2.3.2:240; Thought is typeset as 'Thought' in *The Story of Life*). But the universe that is mind is every bit as tangible and real as what's outside mind because mind experiences its own Thought the same way it experiences another's (*SOL* § 2.1–2.2:393–395). In a sense, the 'tangible' universe of matter–Energy from the self's perspective can be thought of as just another 'mind' that's open to all. We misconceive tangibility because we misconceive life as simply physical and sensorial instead of mental (Thought-based) and awareness–experiential.

Physical Embodiment

Why are you a physically born person at all? The simple reason is that your physical parents, descended from their physical ancestors reaching back to humanity's first generation on Earth nearly 50,000 years ago, physically conceived you (*SOL* § 2:542) in the same way that someone who's Mexican, Japanese, Senegalese, or mixed were conceived by those parents. You are also *physicospirit*. This means you're both physical *and* spirit embodied rather than only spirit embodied as are the spirit-born (SOL § 1.2.1.1.2:249; SOL § 1.1:520) because physicospirit parents conceived you. Even so, and except to the degree you choose to be, you are neither physical *nor* spirit embodied but unique, absolutely autonomous *unembodied* Life, which is to say, *mind* (SOL § 2.1.1.5:353).

Seeing yourself intrinsically physical, that life is only what your body's senses report to your brain, is *your* mindset not human reality. Those who astral project, lucid dream, or interact with spirit persons have awareness–experience of this broader physicospirit reality even if they don't comprehend its scope. Those who don't can discern this reality by mastering energy testing (ET) in the context of an ET community and developing their mind–brain integration to access their spirit senses (SOL § 2:625; *The Big Healing* (TBH; McKeon 2024) CH. 12:165).

Now, there's no such human thing as *physical* life. There's only *physicospirit* life. The reason is twofold. First, the human body is empowered to integrate—entangle—Human. It's not an organism having life on its own terms, independently, as a highly evolved primate. All by itself, without integrating Human, your body is *proto-human*. An animal, not a person. A Living force *entity*, not a Life force *being*. Living means an entity that's 'alive' absent having Life (Living is typeset as 'Living' in *The Story of Life*). Living force is an expression of proto-energy. Life force is the expression of emergent proto-life emanating from the self-aware proto-energy person. This is why the proto-human lifespan averages only 23 years. Absent the integrated person, your body that's empowered to integrate Life is like an airplane sans pilot: it's bound to crash. (Life and Living are further discussed in CH. 1 LIFE FORCE:5; CH. 2 § 2.3.1:50; CH. 2 § 3.2:59; SOL § 2:114; SOL § 2.3.2.1:241; SOL § 1.2:246; SOL § 1.3:272.) When you sever your physicospirit integration, your physical body necessarily dies over the period that your Life force in it dissipates. This is the reason behind death by heartbreak or the loss of the will to live. Physical life is animal. Physicospirit Life is Human.

Second, when Life emergently births as a result of physical (or spirit) conception, it does so with a self-manifested spirit body. This is the natural way of Human birth (SOL § 1.2.1.1.1–1.2.1.1.2:248–249). Physical humans are physicospirit Human. There's no separating spirit from physical embodiment and remaining physically alive. *This is physicospirit*. This is your physical existence as it actually is.

*L*ife as absolutely autonomous means that you, the person, have complete control over your experience. We've heretofore believed that we're doomed to whatever state we're physically born into or encounter throughout our lives. This is inaccurate, the result of a mindset that mind is brain and physical reality the only reality regardless our enduring sense of eternal mind and matter's temporality. You can change your physical appearance right down to your sex because nature doesn't control your genome. You do, in integrating your body (*SOL* § 2.1.3:543). Not simply in the way a driver controls a vehicle, integrating it via the driver's seat the way humans use neural interfaces to control their Na'vi avatars on Pandora in Hollywood's *Avatar* (2009). Rather, since your whole mind integrates your whole body, it's in terms of every aspect of your body responding to mind, from driving it *Avatar*-style to intricately controlling its fundamental physical (DNA) expression.

Imagine climbing into your car and as soon as you integrate it by sitting in the driver's seat, turning it on and touching the steering wheel and foot pedals, it takes on how you want it to look, to be, to perform. You do this subconsciously all day every day with your body via Intentionality. As noted in CH. 1 EMERGENT PROTO-ENERGY on page 3, this means exerting your Thought, meaning thinking–feeling, into the world, into reality. Except the outcome isn't instant. It takes time because the body is a biological entity constituted of matter–Energy. It has its own independently-operating physical reality in the context of the energies of the physical universe, fundamental force, and the 'energy' of the Energent. The latter is the fundamental *existent*—a thing that exists—and the expression of proto-energy in our universe. In *The Story of Life* we call the foregoing applied energy E, real energy Υ (pronounced Upsilon), and proto-energy, respectively. Keep in mind that 'energy' in single quotes always denotes proto-energy or aspects of it, which isn't physical universe energy (e.g., electromagnetic; *SOL* § 1:112–§ 2:114).

Matter bonds and interacts only in accord with its contextual forces. To alter these forces, interactions, and outcomes requires contextually utilizing them Intentionally. Unlike us and depending on how fundamental the change, spirit persons Intentionally alter their spirit bodies at will. The reason is that, unlike *matter* as matter–Energy resisting Intentionality in some way analogous to a gyroscope resisting aspect change, *supramatter*—spirit 'matter' as opposed to physical matter (*SOL* § 1.1:466–§ 1.2:467)—has no independently operating forces controlling it. All equivalent physical forces in the spirit environment readily respond to Intentionality. The spirit person can, for instance, avoid gravity at will because in spirit world gravity is a human-Intentionalized 'force,' not a naturally existing one with its own independent Way of Being as it is in our physical environment.

Your spirit body is a *direct* expression of mind. It is Intentionalized by your mind in the context of human-*dependent* supramatter. Your physical body is an *indirect* expression of mind. It is Intentionalized by your mind in the context of human-*independent* matter–Energy. Where a spirit person can immediately Intentionalize, say, sexual appearance from one sex to the other at will, a physical person needs Intentionalize the same change in the biological context of genome, which initially Intentionalized and habituated as male or female from one's emergent birth (SOL § 2.1.5.1:313).

The reason people show the effects of aging, lifestyle, or stress isn't from shortening telomeres (what science calls programmed cell death), toxic foods, lack of sleep, excess hormonal production, or the inevitable outcome of life. It's because humanity's mindset accepts these effects, which they've observed in animals, as inexorably real for humans. Over time, we subconsciously Intentionalize them at the genomic, hormonal, and other biologically fundamental levels to make them a physical reality in our body. Science, studiously ignoring all aspects of human mind and spirit reality, then presumptively observes them to be causative. This doesn't mean that if one believes something is true then it's a self-fulfilling prophecy. Conscious belief doesn't automatically entail subconscious Intentionality, as it's less powerful in the sense of insistence than the latter. We cover Intentionality in Chapter 6.

Physical human conception isn't the moment the sperm penetrates the egg or the zygote forms. It is that moment in mitosis when a new emergent ℒife births 'in' Energent proto-life. This is *you* when your parents conceived you. Each of us *physicospiritually* embodies as emergent self-aware proto-energy, where proto-energy is a sort of intangibly 'pure' energy and the *Energent* is the expression of proto-energy in our universe whereas *Energent–prime* is the expression of proto-energy in All Existence. Keep these terms in mind as they crop up often in the text. Being physicospirit means that we integrate a physical body while also manifesting a spirit body. Our physical–spirit duality lets us simultaneously experience the natural (physical) and supranatural (spirit) environments of our universe (SOL § 7.1:212).

Mind–brain integration (MBI) means your ethereal ℒife mind integrating your brain such that it instantiates a facsimile of your ℒife mind. This allows it to interact with and experience the physical world. Ideally, MBI is lossless with respect to awareness–experience twixt our physical and spirit realities with no difference in our physical-self and spirit-self personalities.

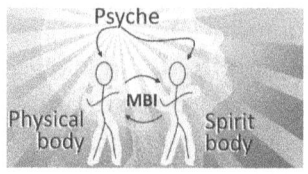

Fig. 1.1. Psyche is spirit embodiment integrating the physical via mind–brain integration along with mind—body integration (CH. 2 § 5:79). Subconscious is stronger than conscious for the physical person and vice versa for the spirit person due to The Corruption (*see* page 12).

What we experience in the one, we have awareness of in the other. The spirit isn't hidden from the physical.

When a physical person dies, he or she continues seamlessly interacting with the supranatural environment via the spirit embodiment he or she has had since conception. For the newly dead physical person, his or her physically alive conscious awareness simply transitions to their conscious spirit awareness and their spirit self feels—has awareness of—their physical body's cessation and the reality of their physical death. There is no 'waking up' from physical life in spirit world nor 'sleeping' in the grave till some judgement day. There is only your conscious ℒife mind integrating your physically instantiated mind having awareness of your physical existence, then having awareness that it has dropped away (in death) and you're now aware of the reality of your spirit-only existence.

The so-called dead aren't intrinsically invisible to our physical selves when we enjoy full mind–brain integration absent the effects of *The Corruption* (CH. 1 THE CORRUPTION on page 12). Ultimately, our physical body integrates our spirit senses and we experience our singular mind in both environments (*Fig. 1.1*).

Death is the *body's* 𝕃iving end, not the infinite *person's* ℒife end. Death's problem lies only in physical separation from the alive and their activities. Yet, physical–spirit separation isn't our emergent Way of Being (*SOL* § 2.2.1.1:234). It's a Corruption of the absolute human autonomy with which Mina Intentionalized our universe as a home for his descendants—*us*—to experience our core essence of ℌuman Way of Being. And that's all a universe really is: a home for a builder's descendants and any others who spiritually immigrate from the megaverse (CH. 2 § 2.1.1:35).

Let's consider how ℒife—you—is transcendent and into where exactly it is that you're emergently birthing and what it means for you. In this book,

Transcendence of ℒife

transcendent means "to be prior to, beyond, and above . . . the universe or material existence" (*Merriam*, s.v. 'transcend; transcendent'). Energent–prime proto-energy is the *fundamental motivating presence* of All Existence, or 'all there infinitely is.' It's the same proto-energy as the Energent of our universe and from which Mina Intentionally built our universe as a human-created aspect of All Existence.

Anything in All Existence *with presence*—having existence—is either proto-energy itself or rooted in it; matter, for instance. The reason is that, ultimately, all existents arise 'in' and of Energent–prime. Energent proto-life is a *L*ife-precursor proto-energy. This is the case because it's a proto-energy having a particular Way of Being that emergently arose from Energent–prime, itself having a unique, emergent Way of Being which led directly to *L*ife's emergent birth.

Emergent *L*ife—you—being a completely different class of presence from Energent–prime, is itself proto-energy. Even so, it isn't Energent–prime nor Energent proto-life because it is *self-aware beingness* having Intentionality. Thus, *L*ife is unique. While Energent–prime is the fundamental *presence* of All Existence, *L*ife is its fundamental *Intentionality*. Of any proto-energy—Energent–prime of All Existence, Energent proto-life, the Energent of our universe—only *L*ife possesses and actualizes Intentionality. It transcends all proto-energy not its own. It might seem this must exclude 'all there infinitely is' since it derives from Energent–prime proto-energy, but Energent–prime and All Existence aren't the same. The former is the *nature* of All Existence and the latter the *reality* of proto-energy that grounds in it. *L*ife necessarily is part of 'all there infinitely is,' yet transcends all aspects of it (sol § 5:294; sol § 1:303).

Since *L*ife transcends 'all there infinitely is,' it's not beholden to it the way a universe (matter) is. Neither first-emergence *L*ife (described in ch. 2) nor subsequently Intentionalized *L*ife (all of us) is locked into any particular spatial location, universe, or embodiment. Mind integrating body transcends it. Whereas you being born into a physical body indeed ties you to it for the duration of your physical life, your mind is free to range far and wide from its spatial (embodied) location in our universe. We're not talking astral projection (sol § 1:591) or imagination but *mind awareness*. This is the state in which you shift your conscious awareness—recall that *L*ife emerges into beingness 'in' Energent proto-life where your discrete self exists wherever its awareness is at any given moment (sol § 2.3.2:240)—from your physical body to any other environment such as the supranatural (spirit) environment or humanity's original unembodied Energent proto-life environment (sol § 1.2.1:247).

For us here on Earth having limited mind–brain integration (sol § 1.2.2.5:261) and lacking an understanding of reality as well as any practice in the art, literally shifting our conscious awareness to a place other than where our physical body resides seems fantastical. But for those in the supranatural environment having both an understanding of reality and practice in the art, Intentionality (which does involve a certain imaginative focus) is sufficient to shift one's conscious awareness from point A to B. And because their spirit body Intentionalizes from mind then their spirit body naturally manifests wherever their awareness resides. We can't do that with our physical body (*Star Trek*'s transporters notwithstanding) because it's a physical existent with its own independent Way of Being. Since you, being physically alive, are physicospirit, you constantly interact with your own spirit self as well as spirit reality regardless how spiritually obtuse or in denial you practically may be. This mode of being empowers constant interaction with spirit reality according to your mind–brain integration-empowered conscious awareness and subconscious awareness.

The bottom line is that you are not your body. You, the person, the emergently self-aware proto-energy being—*Life*—don't exist *in* or *as* your physical body nor even your spirit body, but transcendently 'in' Energent proto-life. Your emergent birth (conception of *Life* not of your physical body) simply shifted your self-awareness to where your body was—in the womb, since you were physically conceived—and that's what *integration* is. Consequently, we think it's inevitable and that physical embodiment is our only existence. Well, it's neither. And, being transcendent of physicospirit embodiment, All Existence is your oyster.

Mina built our universe with Intentionality. It was not magical, deific, or emergent. It was a human endeavor... Intentionality is intrinsic of

The Corruption

the human person, the self-aware proto-energy self. *The Story of Life* explains why and how one of Mina's own sisters, a universe builder herself, Intentionalized *The Corruption* into our universe (SOL § 2:367). We don't get into its details here, but it's sufficient to say that The Corruption is her addicting universal humanity to a mindset we call *Accountableism*. Her purpose with physical humanity was to degrade our mind–brain integration to enthrall us to materialism—that our beingness is physical not physicospirit—as a nonautonomous mode of existence to keep us unaware of absolute autonomy, which Mina built into the 'energy' of his *Life* force entangling the person. Her interference was predicated on her and other universe builders' belief that absolute autonomy is detrimental to megaversal humanity, i.e., all humans in all human-built universes (CH. 2 § 2.1.1:35).

In practical terms, The Corruption is *mindset addiction* to a Way of Being of Accountableism, which results in a Way of Being of nonautonomy that's seemingly without choice. The reason for this state of affairs doesn't lie in megalomania, evil, power, control, greed, so-called human nature, some Way of Being arising in All Existence ('all there infinitely is'), or the like. Quite unexpectedly, it rises in *altruism* which essence, ostensibly, is to do no harm. Accountableism as altruism was Mina's sister's way to remove the absolute autonomy of spirit-born humanity, whereas degrading mind–brain integration to a level of total unawareness of our physicospirit reality was her way to remove the absolute autonomy of physical-born humanity. This is why the physical-born—you and me—have until now had no awareness of the 'energy' of ℒife force. This lack of awareness translates to a lack of choice that's intrinsic of absolute autonomy such that physical humanity became addicted to the mindset of physical frailty as our one and only reality of physical existence.

Altruism took firmer root in the physical environment than the spirit one where mind–brain integration was degraded and life appeared random, tenuous, and, above all, entirely physical with a concomitant determination to preserve it despite any belief in a glorious afterlife. The physical-born came to associate harm with universal truths of wrongness, badness, and evil, the avoidance of which they associated with the highest good and thus a virtue. In adopting this standard, however, they substituted a faux Way of Being rooted in nonautonomy for their core emergent Way of Being rooted in absolute autonomy (SOL § 1:361). In this, contradiction and self-conflict arose; the sense that we're just not right, somehow broken, at odds with creation and our creator. Altruism necessarily inflicts harm ostensibly to prevent harm. It's therefore self-negating. It can never solve human suffering regardless how rapturous philosophy is of it. It's The Corruption because it corrupts our core Way of Being for which our minds ceaselessly strive.

The Corruption made physical–spirit separation our chief experience not only of death but of life, too (SOL § 1:361; SOL § 2.3:545). We correspondingly built the mindset that death is a fixture of life, a permanent separation twixt the living and the dead regardless afterlife beliefs. Real faith in life after death should mourn only death's temporary separation than the loss of life it appears. But few have this mindset, partly owing to fear. Their subconscious roots only in what's materially observable while studiously ignoring what's immaterial, which is only *less* observable.

The Negative Collective Consciousness (NCC; SOL § 4.2.1.4:382) was, until 2017, an 'energy' field of negative emotive ℒife force (EmℒF; referring to the concept of emotive energy) suffusing our universe just as Energent proto-energy does. Proto-energy's natural Way of Being is 'neutral' (not as in applied energy E; SOL § 1.1:392). Mind as an aspect of the self-aware proto-energy person is, accordingly, also fundamentally 'neutral' subconscious proto-energy in full interactive contact with Energent proto-energy thus EM𝓛F. Mind therefore experienced the 'energy' of the NCC the way, say, an empath experiences the emotive energy (EM𝓛F) of others. This is why, throughout history, no person could successfully overcome so-called human nature. It's the origin on Earth of our concept of sin.

<small>The Negative Collective Consciousness</small>

Humanity Intentionalized the NCC into existence out of 'neutral' proto-energy over time via Thought rooted in the mindset of The Corruption. Its presence Intentionally influenced each person's mindset with its negative 'energy' in the same way a person Intentionalizes Thought proto-energy around individuals to foment particular mindstate responses, like a vibe that darkens a person's feelings. This happens because mind is exquisitely sensitive to it. It's why negative EM𝓛F can shift one's mood. It affected all 𝓛ife force, 𝕃iving–𝓛ife force (human body), and 𝕃iving force entities of the natural environment.

Mina could never compete with the NCC, as it arose from humanity and permeated the universe and every mind within it the way a stink permeates every nostril exposed to it. He couldn't simply re-Intentionalize it as a big, bad, universe builder. It belonged to humanity, his descendants, who created it. Only humanity, the creator of the NCC, could collectively neutralize its proto-energy back to its normative, 'neutral' state. Any individual could have albeit ineffectually done this because each individual is a part of the overall Intentionality.

Jesus by himself could have done so by dint of his full awareness of human spirit reality (more than any other besides Mina, that is; *see* Jesus' testimony in SOL § 1.3.3.2:475). He didn't because, without so-called archangel Michael and Lucifer reconciling, the Ultraculture fueling humanity's mindset would have remained in place save for a momentary change in mindstate that people would feel like an inexplicable mood blip if they felt anything at all. So, while an individual *could* neutralize the NCC, it wouldn't last longer than about half a picosecond. In conversation with Mina, Jesus waited in the hope that Michael and Lucifer would reconcile to deliver a real end to the NCC, as finally happened with their Reconciliation October 13, 2017 as a spontaneous re-Intentionalization by universal humanity (*TBH*, SOL CH. 4; SOL CH. 40 Jesus:613; SOL § 4.2.1–4.2.2.2:379–384).

1 The Universe in Which You Live

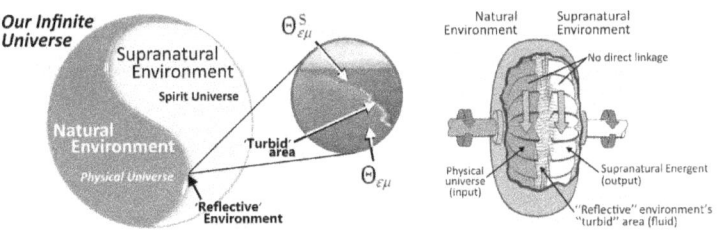

Fig. 1.2. Left, exploded view of the environments of our infinite universe; 'turbid' area is the proximal interaction of the natural and supranatural Energents in the 'reflective' environment. Right, a basic automatic transmission (fluid coupler) conceptualized as a process that bridges the natural and supranatural environments to indirectly translate *enérgeia* (CH. 2 § 3.3.3.1:68).

Side Note. Michael and Lucifer embodied The Corruption in their Accountableist conflict more than any others. 'Angels' don't exist. Such beings are spirit-born humans. Satan isn't a being but a myth that Michael inflicted on his brother (SOL § 4:377; § 2:522).

Our infinite universe is a wholistic, physicospirit structure composed of two interwoven and fully interactive environments, the natural and supranatural. Philosophy with a capital-P (representing all types of inquiry as humanity's primary knowledge-seeking class of study) generally renders these as the physical and spirit worlds (*Fig. 1.2, left*). While the natural–supranatural is indeed a fundamental demarcation, they meet in a 'reflective' environment where a 'turbid' proto-energy area forms a 'fluid' bridge between the two Energents (*Fig. 1.2, right*; recall, single-quoting terms incl. 'frequency,' 'density,' etc. is a convention to help visualize their discrete similitude).

A physicospirit person (*you*) exists simultaneously in all three of these discrete yet interconnected environments—four, if you include consciousness (psyche)—as a singular, wholistic entity. If our physicospirit senses integrated as intended, then when we looked in the mirror (so to speak) we'd be able to perceive our physical body here in the natural environment, our body's nonphysical 'reflection' in the 'reflective' environment, and our spirit body in the supranatural environment. All three are aspects of your embodiment as a self-aware proto-energy person, a conscious being. The natural environment is sufficiently self-explanatory, and we don't further describe it here. Bear in mind, though, that it includes both the physical *and* 'reflective' environments as a wholistic integration.

The 'Reflective' (non-Physical) Environment. Everything in the natural environment down to its fundamental archí—the cardinal unit of matter—'reflects' in the 'reflective' environment. This means that physical matter has two apparent forms: physical and nonphysical (*note, however, that nonphysical is* not *the same as spirit*). The nonphysical 'reflective' is too ethereal for our physical senses to experience, as its proto-energy is less 'energy dense' than the physical. It has no purpose as such; it's more an artifact of the way the natural and supranatural Energents behave and interact. As an interface, it bridges the difference between the natural and supranatural environments (*Fig. 1.2, right*). Chakras, for instance, are Intentionalized by Mina as a purposed phenomenon of this 'reflective' environment (SOL CH. 29:497). They serve to bridge physical and spirit persons so they can interact despite degraded mind–brain integration.

The 'reflective' environment isn't a real environment the way the physical and spirit environments are real. It's more a boundary between the natural and supranatural Energents. The supranatural environment is *reactive* in proximity to the phenomena (motion and force) of the natural one. Its reaction to these is what gives rise to the 'turbidity' of the proto-energy in the 'reflective.' The phenomena's 'turbid' effect is that it composites dimensional physical motion—a moving car, a tree, a living cell right on down to singular archí oscillations—into a dimensionless (neither physical nor spirit) 'reflection' of physical matter and its applied energy E phenomena. Think of a mirror as an analogue where the physical world 'reflects' as a mirror image. This is the 'reflective.' Everything in it exists three-dimensionally and is in motion just as in the actual physical environment. The difference is that, as with a real mirror, the *forces* in the physical world only 'reflect' as already exerted expressions. If you touch a mirrored flame, say, you don't feel the heat, you don't get burned. Unlike a two-dimensional mirror, the 'reflective' environment is a three-dimensional environment. A spirit person there is fully immersed as if inside Harry Potter's magic mirror where they see and experience the *forces* of the physical world but not the *effects*—heat, wind, wetness—of those forces.

The 'reflective' environment appears real because it's a fully dimensional representation of physical matter and its applied energy E phenomena. And, yet, it's *not* those things. *It's just a 'reflection,' an effect of the 'energy' of matter-Energy.* The physical world is dynamic—has dynamism—because fundamental force is real in the physical environment. Flame produces heat. Heat causes change in matter. The 'reflective' environment is nondynamic. It has no dynamism apart from its physical counterpart any more than a shadow has apart from what cast it. A spirit person visiting the natural environment can only perceive and (with Intentionality) interact with this 'reflection,' not with the physical world itself. This is how spirit persons interact with the physical world.

For example, when it appears to us that a spirit person is manipulating a physical, meaning a material, object—say, a light switch—they're actually moving its 'reflection' via Intentionalized 'energy,' not via their spirit hands. Such movement in the 'reflective' necessarily translates to some degree to the physical object. This moves the physical entity since the 'reflective' and physical object integrate like a shadow with what cast it. When a structurally sound physical building collapses for no discernible reason, it's occasionally because spirit persons undermined its support (often by Intentionally increasing its load beyond what's expected from physical matter like snow and ice) in the 'reflective.' A partial or full collapse necessarily follows.

Spirit persons in the 'reflective' experience physical reality going about its business all around them as though *in* the physical world, but they're actually experiencing its nonphysical 'reflection.' They can't see or experience the actually physical because its 'energy density' is beyond the limits of their spirit senses similar to the way certain high or low frequencies are beyond the limits of our physical senses. Since physical matter's applied energy E phenomena 'reflects' there, too, then a spirit person (who isn't a 'reflected' part of this environment) experiences its *phenomena*—rain, wind, fire— just as a physical person does. But they don't experience its *effect* such as wetness, blowing hair, and burns. This is because the phenomena isn't real. It's a 'reflection.'

A spirit person can walk through a 'reflected' wall because the 'energy density' of their spirit body is less than that of the 'reflected' wall. They feel the sensation of it scraping as they pass through but aren't scraped because its 'energy density' isn't sufficiently 'dense.' They feel the raindrops falling through their body but aren't wetted. They feel wind on their skin but no heating or cooling effect. Their hair doesn't blow around. All this because their spirit body isn't as 'energy dense' as the 'reflective' environment, which itself isn't as 'energy dense' as the physical one (*SOL* § 7.2.1.2:217). The 'reflective' environment, which is filled with spirit persons, is what the physically alive experience when they astral project.

The proto-energy of the 'reflective' is that of the supranatural (spirit) Energent. It 'flows through' from the supranatural environment to the 'reflective' one. But, in so doing, it takes on a greater 'energy density' than what the supranatural Energent has as a function of its proximity to archí oscillations—from quantum particles to stars—in the context of the 'reflective.' However, it is significantly less 'energy dense' than the natural (physical) Energent. In other words, the supranatural Energent's 'energy density' becomes greater in the context of the 'reflective' environment as an effect of its reaction to physical-world archí motion. But remember that all apparent dynamism—the actual forces involved in molecular and atomic motion—in the 'reflective' is only a 'reflection' of the *effect* of physical forces in the physical world. On its own, the 'reflective' is a nondynamic environment. There are no physical world forces exerting energy in the 'reflective.'

Any physical entity, right down to its constituent archí, 'reflects' in the 'reflective' aspect of the natural–supranatural Energent so long as it physically exists. Also, what seem like extra or inexplicable animal senses, or aspects of human sixth sense, are in part 'reflective-self' phenomena. These arise in the chakras, a 'reflective' aspect of the 'reflective' body that translates 'energy' there into our physical bodies. Only humans and certain companion animals (e.g., dogs, cats, horses; *SOL* CH. 39:601) have dynamism in the 'reflective' environment because these alone integrate autonomous spirit bodies (*SOL* § 1:303) distinct from their 'reflective' bodies. A physical person who's spirit-aware and trained can consciously interact via their spirit body with any nondynamic 'reflective' object—human bodies, animals, bugs, bacteria, DNA, inanimate objects—as well as the dynamic spirit body of other persons, certain companion animals, and spirit world residents.

The Supranatural Spirit Environment. Matter in the supranatural environment, which we call supramatter, differs fundamentally from natural matter just as its Energent differs from the natural Energent. This difference is why we can't physically interact with supramatter using our physical body. We need our 'reflective self' as a bridge via the chakras to integrate our brain–body with mind's awareness of the supranatural (*aware* in the sense that our mind integrates our brain more than the current normal). When we're brain aware—this refers to our physically instantiated mind—of the supranatural, we can consciously interact with that environment using our spirit body even while physically alive and awake. This is how (legit) mediums consciously experience spirit persons. Mina provided for our complete freedom of existence—our full, absolutely autonomous Way of Being—in the way he structured our universe and physical embodiment. When we understand how reality works, we are quite unlimited in what we can be, do, feel, and experience.

All things need energy to exist. From stars to rocks to things alive, energy holds it all together and enlivens it. This means the Energent that creates archí and binds it into forms like stars and planets from which sunlight, air, water, and so forth arise to support physical life. That's all separate and apart from *vital*

How the Physical Powers the Spirit

energy—Living and ℒife force—that enlivens things, makes them actually *alive*. Living force comes to entities through their 'reflected' body's chakras via the natural Energent (*SOL* CH. 29:497; every nonhuman entity has at least one chakra). ℒife force is human. It comes to our physical body via integrating our emergent ℒife self.

Our spirit body isn't *exactly* a body in the physical sense, meaning an objective existence in its own right—an existent—with independent processes and mechanisms that requires self-maintenance. Rather, it's a manifestation of mind without need of conscious Thought. Our mind just does it. It coalesces from proto-energy via subconscious Intentionality into spirit matter—supramatter—having human form. Perhaps the easiest way to picture this is to imagine how you see yourself in your mind's eye without any conscious wishful thinking. Are you tall, short, good looking, ugly, happy, bright, sour, dull, dynamic, having gravitas, undignified, or whatever? In the same way that you physically walk around projecting a natural or contrived self-image, the intrinsic capability of your mind to integrate supranatural 'energy' naturally manifests your spirit body into real supranatural form.

The 'energy' we're talking about here is Energent proto-energy. But it can't directly translate to the supranatural Energent the way that Energent–prime 'flows' into the natural Energent of our universe like an ocean into a bay. This is because the natural Energent is an organic expression of emergent Energent–prime whereas the supranatural Energent is a universe builder's own Intentional creation. It is substantively different. We call it (supranatural) *Energent* because it serves the same functional purpose, but it's a human-built construct, a facsimile. It's not an organic expression of Energent–prime, the root of All Existence, nor an aspect of the 'energy' of 'all there infinitely is.' Operational incompatibility between the natural and supranatural Energents arises from this substantive difference. The result is different operational symmetries (in the sense of invariance).

The natural Energent, like its emergent Energent–prime parent, is non-transformable absent an emergence event. But the supranatural Energent is, because its Way of Being is Intentionally invariant absent Intentional change by its builder. Take, for example, an ocean cline where waters don't mix. As properties like temperature, density, and salinity equalize (convert), such initially immiscible waters necessarily integrate (*Fig. 1.2* on page 15 (inset), *left*). *Enérgeia* similarly converts to a supranaturally integrable norm. *Enérgeia* is 'energy.' It's the Energent's *expression* in time and space, recalling that the Energent itself has no time and space and is the proto-energy inside the archí constituting its entirety (SOL § 6.11.4:198). The reason for conversion—translation—is straightforward.

Mina built the supranatural Energent with Intentionality whereas the natural Energent is an organic expression—an appendage—of Energent–prime. It has unique, adjunctive properties but isn't encapsulated, or segregated, from All Existence. He Intentionalized—guaranteed—our universe to interface with it. The natural Energent is discrete yet wholistic vis-à-vis Energent–prime. While the supranatural environment is singularly one of 'energy' in which supramatter arises only in response to Intentionality, the natural environment is one of mixed matter–Energy. In the context of a universe, matter—archí—emergently arises from proto-energy with its own existentiality, or independent Way of Being, that constructs complex forms of its own accord.

The supranatural environment needs 'energy' to exist in the same way the natural environment does. However, the supranatural Energent doesn't manufacture 'energy' because it's not a real Energent. It's only an Intentionalized facsimile. Thus, it's a net 'energy' *consumer*. It consumes the 'energy' of the natural Energent that's an aspect of Energent–prime, the fundamental proto-energy of All Existence, or 'all there infinitely is.' Therefore, the natural Energent is a real Energent that, in the context of the natural environment, manufactures 'energy' via certain physical processes. Accordingly, it's a net 'energy' *producer*. The upshot is that the supranatural Energent must import its 'energy' from the natural Energent.

How does conversion and importation occur? Well, pretty simply. In brief, 'energy' translation begins in the natural environment. *Translation* is a term that describes the movement of 'energy' without motion. This is different from energy moving through space in the physical universe via wave and other motion. Translation begins with single pairwise archí in motion that 'reflects' *as if* motion in the supranatural environment, where translation ends. The 'energy' of the physical pairwise archí is now supranatural 'energy' that's available to sustain the supranatural environment. Spirit persons Intentionally use this 'energy' for their daily lives, including to manifest their spirit bodies as tangible supramatter. How this process happens isn't germane to this book, but you can read *The Story of Life* for details on the three methods that accomplish this task (SOL § 7.1.3:214–7.5:222).

You don't come into human existence as a physically conceived creature nor have existence in and of your physical body as does nonhuman life. Physical conception triggers your emergent birth as a human person 'in' a proto-energy environment that we call Energent proto-life. This is what you are as a being. Not physical matter. Not amorphous spirit. Not the mere thought of God. You're an 'energy' being that experiences 'energy' and that's all.

Summary of Chapter 1

Your emergent self-aware proto-energy self—the *you* that is you—Intentionalizes your subconscious–conscious mind in this milieu. You integrate its Way of Being with your physical body having its own independent Way of Being. It serves as an interface, or 'avatar,' to interact with the natural (physical) environment of our universe. Your self-aware proto-energy self manifests your spirit body in the supranatural (spirit) environment at emergent birth out of human-dependent supramatter (spirit world matter). It manifests only your emergent Way of Being and is a supramaterial extension of your mind to interact with the supranatural environment of our universe. These two embodiments give you full access to every jot and tittle of our wholistic universe as a physicospirit person having a full, simultaneous experience of these physical and spirit environments.

Accordingly, your physical body is not flesh and blood that's out of your control. It's under your mind's absolute command, from its genetic bits to the whole shebang. You are not condemned to biological interference with your health. You don't exist as an animal with all the realities that we observe in the natural world. And that's the point of all the metaphysical talk here: to paint you a different picture of your existence in this world than you've hitherto believed or imagined so that you might discover the real keys to physical health and wellbeing not to mention psyche (mind) healing. We call this *healing through awareness*.

The next chapter is a more detailed overview of 1) what your body is, 2) the origin of humanity in All Existence and the body's physical origin, 3) the milieu in which your body lives, 4) your mind and body as a physicospirit unit, 5) the infinity of self (psyche), and 6) the meaning of Way of Being.

This book may seem a daunting read filled with new and unusual concepts that challenge much if not all that you believe. Yet, comprehending your reality in the world you inhabit is an important prerequisite to gaining control over your physical health and wellbeing. Don't be concerned if you don't absorb it all to your satisfaction in the first or even subsequent reads. The important thing is that your subconscious is gaining awareness and will begin working on its own regardless any conscious confusion you may feel.

Your Body — Christopher McKeon

How Your Body Works in Our Universe

The information in this chapter may not feel philosophically or religiously sound according to your worldview. And it isn't necessary for you to experience physical healing by a healer nor to impart at least some healing into your body yourself as you gain awareness of your physicospirit existence. This chapter is, however, quite necessary to help free your mind of the belief that you're just a brain in a body in a material world. That that's all you are. That you're chained to the natural, living world which you—your thought—can't affect any more than wishful thinking. That you're no more than a blade of grass in a meadow that can't avoid biology's grazing teeth to change your physical reality one iota.

Such beliefs short-circuit your ability to exert full (beyond what humanity has always presumed as 'natural') healing in your body. This is because, in your deepest thoughts, you believe it's an impossibility. You then turn to your favorite philosophical or religious belief to justify it and reassure yourself. This chapter asks you to suspend your ingrained, habituated beliefs to fairly consider a different take on yourself, your body, your world, your universe . . . on 'all there infinitely is.'

So, forget about your brain and genetics controlling your mind, body, self . . . your very life. That's all a red herring by those having no certainty outside uninformed observation while rejecting the broader palette of human experience and what motivates the human body to *life* and the self to *beingness*.

Because you, my friend, are a *being*, not a body.

A *mind*, not a brain.

A *person*, not a smarter animal.

Absolutely autonomous, not the slave, servant, child, or creation of anyone or anything.

Your physical body is an integration through which you, a mind, can phenomenally experience an environment outside your mind. *Integration* means that your psyche—your mind, your consciousness, your fundamental self howsoever you imagine it—doesn't merely *inhabit* your body but *amalgamates* it so thoroughly that, in essence, it's an extension of your mind.

Yes, your body exists here on Earth (in the spirit environment, too; read *The Story of Life* for those details). Your mind, however, exists everywhere as *awareness*. Although your mind is present as reality where your body is, it can be present as reality—as awareness—anywhere. You don't exist in or as your physical body but transcendently 'in' what *The Story of Life* calls Energent proto-life. Your mind simply shifts its awareness into your physical body and *that's* integration. It happens naturally and without conscious awareness during conception, meaning at your emergent birth 'in' Energent proto-life. Consequently, we think our physically alive awareness is inevitable and physical embodiment our only existence. It's neither. Accordingly, you are not your body. You are your mind. More fundamentally, you are self-aware proto-energy. An *emergent proto-energy being*. This is what people are trying to get at when they say the human person is energy, not matter. It means that, in the context of your physical body, your mind is all powerful. In control. Making your body what it is.

This chapter gives you a comprehensive overview of where your physical body comes from and the milieu in which it exists, as they're inseparable. This necessarily includes where humanity itself comes from; the fundamental structure and energies of existence of which humanity, therefore you, are a part; your mind and body; the concept of Way of Being; and Intentionality, which is your mind's ability to exert Thought into reality as transformational 'energy.'

It's an important chapter because, in order to effectually transform your body and keep it in a state of undiminished health, it's necessary that you have a reasonable understanding of what your body is and how it exists. You can't do that without understanding where it comes from, the milieu in which it operates, and how the person that is you exists as emergent *Life* in this world in which you live. Because, ultimately, it's your emergent birth *as* ℒife that makes you what you are, having the ability to heal your body. Read *The Story of ℒife* for greater detail.

Section 1
What Is the Body

First things first: you don't exist merely as a physical body here on planet Earth. If you already believe you're transcendent of your body then consider that you weren't created into existence by some Higher Power. You don't exist as a vague entity 'out there.' Or in the bosom of God. As amorphous spirit over and above or better than physicality. You are mind, to be sure. You are also, and fundamentally, a 'self-aware proto-energy being.' This means that, in your very essence which transcends even mind, you're of the same 'energy' as All Existence (*below*). Except that, unlike it, you're self-aware thus having ℒife.

If you can imagine our universe in its infinite sense, which is to say indeterminate and dimensionless, then you've formed a working image of what we call All Existence, which is 'all there infinitely is.' This includes the human-created universe that we observe. We've heretofore believed our universe itself to be all there infinitely is. But it's not. Our universe is only one aspect of All Existence. Accordingly, it's as time infinite and existence infinite as All Existence despite having a definable beginning.

Before our universe existed, before our supposed Big Bang, there was All Existence. Before All Existence itself existed... well, All Existence existed. Back through indeterminate timelessness, there was All Existence. It was a *different* All Existence, absolutely. But, being time infinite and existence infinite, it was nonetheless *the* All Existence because there can never be two of 'all there infinitely is' (SOL § 1:100; SOL CH. 16:106). What this means is that All Existence has never not existed even though our universe, an aspect of 'all that infinitely is,' had a start in time approximately 14 billion (Earth) years ago. Today, what we call Current All Existence as the present iteration of 'all there infinitely is' is an emergently 'evolved' *existentiality*—the characteristic of 'existence'—of timeless All Existence.

The idea that existence has always existed is difficult to grasp because we live in simplistic causality fixed around matter where something is always causatively prior to something else. But comprehending it isn't impossible. To grasp your existence and therefore your power to control your physical wellbeing, it's necessary to let go of the causative reality of our universe, of your body and, of course, of you yourself to appreciate the eternal nature of existence thus your own eternal beingness.

All this may feel like a ball of yarn that's unwinding and becoming snarled and, therefore, uncomprehensible. But don't get overwhelmed by the deluge of new terms and ideas. Keep reading as we explain. Your subconscious will take it in, start working with it, and making sense of it. Now, let's consider All Existence in more detail.

1.1 All Existence

All Existence is 'all there infinitely is.' To describe it, one can only say it is *Way of Being* because it's formless, intangible, without time or space. When you grasp All Existence *as* Way of Being, then you comprehend All Existence. It has never not existed although its Way of Being emergently 'evolved' over time. In this respect, it differs fundamentally from our universe. It comes to be as it is via self-organized *emergence* as a first cause along an emergent path from a *previous* All Existence Way of Being to an *emergent* All Existence Way of Being until finalizing as our *current* All Existence Way of Being. This is the All Existence that humanity recognizes today in its imperfect understanding of our universe or, for some, as something more than our universe (*SOL Fig.* 101:233).

All Existence possesses something akin to albeit not exactly like plant-like intelligence. In some ways, it operates like a mind except without sentience–sapience (consciousness–wisdom). It expresses not in any distributed network sense but as *nonconscious* Way of Being via *Energent–prime*, which *The Story of Life* calls fundamental *proto-energy*. The proto-energy of our universe is an aspect of Energent–prime (*SOL* § 1:112).

1.1.1 Emergence Defined

What exactly is emergence? We use the general concept of emergence in the literature as a primer. For example, diverse entities of a system locally disturb, differentiate, and coalesce in novel, coherent structures, "surfacing innovations and distinctions among its parts" (Holman 2010, 14) sufficient to globally disrupt the system. The system itself differentiates and ultimately coalesces—self-assembling and self-organizing—into a novel, coherent system in ways that are, even in principle, irreducible to their emergent constituents. Emergent "even-in-principle irreducibility" (Piiroinen 2014, 146) recognizes that the sum is sometimes more, if not other than, its parts. And, too, that "entities (properties or substances) 'arise' out of more fundamental entities and yet are 'novel' or 'irreducible' with respect to them" (O'Connor et al. 2015, par. 1; *see also*, O'Connor 1994, De Wolf et al. 2005, and Clayton 2006, 1–31).

Such entities are new, surprising, and unpredictable. Author Steven Johnson puts it this way: "[A]gents residing on one scale start producing behavior that lies one scale above them: ants create colonies; urbanites create neighborhoods; simple pattern-recognition software learns how to recommend new books. The movement from low-level rules to higher-level sophistication is... emergence" (2001, 18). They're viewed as *weakly* emergent when they're "*unexpected* given the principles" of their constituent parts (Chalmers 2006, 244, *io*; e.g., cellular automata, "a paradigm of emergence in recent complex systems theory"), or *strongly* emergent when they're "*not deducible* even in principle" from their constituent parts (ibid, *io*; e.g., quantum entanglement). Philosophically, emergence is something from nothing although something never comes from nothing (*SOL* § 2.1.1:231).

"Emergence in human systems has produced new technologies, towns, democracy, and some would say consciousness—the capacity for self-reflection" (Holman, 19). Emergence is the rise of novel, self-organized existence. A first cause. You, yourself, are an emergent being.

1.1.2 Energent–prime Intelligence

In *The Story of Life*, we describe in detail an ontological *grounding unit* system. It explicates how we can understand All Existence today in terms of—*grounding in*—its previous existence; how it was then before it was what it is now. This understanding removes the infinite causal loop problem that Philosophy with a capital-P has. This is the idea that, no matter how far back one goes, there must always and infinitely be yet another cause for existence (*SOL* CH. 15:99). This problem has long stymied philosophy and theology.

In essence, a previous All Existence transcends a series of emergent self-organizations before settling into the stable, coherent, transformationally satisfied final-phase system of a current All Existence. In our case, that would be what we call Current All Existence. It features emergent, unaware nonconscious intelligence that expresses via Energent–prime plus human consciousness which itself emergently births 'in' Energent proto-life. This is how we comprehend time infinity of 'all there infinitely is' without the problem of infinite causal regress that's raised by the clash between causality and eternity never getting to an ultimate starting point.

When we talk about *unaware nonconscious intelligence* (UNI), we're altogether referring to All Existence, Energent–prime, and UNI wholistically and holistically, since all existents—a thing that exists—in All Existence are simultaneously discrete yet equivalent.

> **Side note.** As used throughout, *wholism* is the whole in and of itself—the unified whole; a jigsaw puzzle with its imagery that's all put together. *Holism* is the parts as they interact to create the whole, and the relationship between the parts and whole. The distinction follows from the emergent type, which isn't greater than the sum of its parts so much as transcends the whole that was greater than the sum of *its* parts.

All existents are discrete as a *mode of being* but equivalent as a *mode of existence* (SOL § 8:223). A mode of being means a *logical mode*, the *nature* of Way of Being. A mode of existence means an *existent mode*, *how* Way of Being *operates*. Here, logical mode differs in functionality but is equivalent to existent mode in principle (*note that equivalent in principle doesn't imply the same in principle*). Logical mode is the *way* it is, meaning it's the *reality of existence*, or (the nature of) *reality* in toto. Existent mode is equivalent in functionality but differs in nature from logical mode. It's the *how* it is, meaning it's the *nature of existence*, or (the nature of) how reality *operates* in toto. We develop this interrelatedness farther below.

That said, however, the point we're making here is that UNI in union with All Existence is neither equivalent nor equal to mind in union with body. In other words, All Existence is not some infinite mind–body writ large; the one doesn't exist in terms of the other. That concept is alien.

What UNI is not is sapient or sentient. Current All Existence, inclusive of Energent–prime, isn't a conscious being or a self-regulating organism any more than planet Earth is sentient Gaia (Lovelock 1979).

> **Side Note.** *The Story of Life* notes that Earth indeed is a dynamical system where all parties shape the ecosphere. Through individual functions that are, in aggregate, self-regulatory generally but not as a holistic organism capable of self-regulation, Earth maintains a homeostasis fit for life in the absence of probabilistically inevitable exigencies—asteroids, supervolcanoes, solar crises—and humans who are free to blow it up if they choose.
>
> Mina's underlying causal intent forms the deterministic and emergent activities of the larger natural environment to ensure the only outcome is a biosphere that's fit for life. That outcome is distinct from exigencies also a natural part of the universe and inevitable within Mina's larger, universal causal intent. As humans are eternal beings, it's no sweat for Mina to start over after disaster; he's repeatedly done so (disaster on inhabited planets isn't his original Way of Being of our universe; SOL § 2.2.1:233; SOL CH. 32:531). On the other hand, humans are capable of Intentionally averting disaster (CH. 6 § 2:140).

Rather, Current All Existence is a *quinta essentia* (Latin: *fifth essence* and the root of quintessence in medieval philosophy, hearkening back to an unknown medium bathing All Existence called æther, though currently in science it's known as dark energy) that predates Current All Existence, reaching all the way back to when there was only indeterminate (note: not *indeterminance*). It's not material, spirit, or 'energetic.' Its essence emergently iterated—repeated again and again—such that its iterative environment *now* is no longer how it was *then*. It's a noncognitive essence without consciousness; not a being or a person but more a universal 'subconscious' albeit not in any human or conscious sense. From its existence in Previous All Existence, it emergently self-assembled and self-organized during the aforementioned system-level emergence into its novel and unexpected quintessence in Current All Existence (*see*, e.g., Sahni 2002; Zlatev et al. 1999).

Similar overall to a caterpillar self-digesting into a butterfly—caterpillar is mode of being but *like* a logical mode (reality of existence); caterpillar*ness* is mode of existence but *like* an existent mode (nature of existence)—emergent UNI (the butterfly) is not just more than the sum of its parts (the caterpillar), but transcends the whole (its caterpillarness) that was greater *then* than those *now* non-existent parts. This essence is the source for which science sees an ordered and seemingly designed-for-life universe (e.g., Davies 2007) that, in terms of ℒife, includes—not that Philosophy with a capital-P would ever admit it—physical and spirit environments (SOL § 7.1:212).

UNI is an 'adaptive force' but doesn't rise to ℒife force, the emergent proto-energy that is each one of us. Mina likens it to brainstem intelligence (SOL § 2.2.1.2:237). It's discrete; an individual entity amongst all the entities of All Existence. In one sense, All Existence qualifies as an entity because it has a distinct and objective existence although, dictionarily, it doesn't "exist[s] apart from other things, having its own independent existence" (*Cambridge*, s.v. 'entity'). All Existence is 'all there infinitely is.' Its every entity is an integral, interrelated part of a whole while at the same time free, autonomous, and independent to experience and even change its existence on its own terms in a way that transcends our everyday sense of either wholism or holism.

No part of existence is constrained intrinsically by the whole of existence. Everything in existence that's nonhuman shares in a predilection toward order, congruence, coherence, consistency, and so on which (like freedom, autonomy, and independence) is a self-organized subsystemic trait that permeates the system. That trait is UNI. But don't think intelligence presupposes order or that order presupposes intelligence; it can just as well presuppose disorder or, as indeed it does, nonintelligence from order. Why, then, would Mina pick *intelligence* to describe this nonconscious, noncognitive trait? There are three reasons: Way of Being, existence interface, and traits. We describe Way of Being below, as it's pertinent to this book, and leave existence interface and traits to *The Story of Life* (§ 2.2.1.2:237; § 2.2.1.3:238, respectively).

1.1.3 Way of Being

Briefly, the nature of intelligence is that it *is* Way of Being similar to how All Existence *is* Way of Being. Intelligence itself, its reality, is mainly about how one is, where *how one is* means the totality of an entity relationally with the totality of environment. It's not "the ability to learn, understand, and make judgments or have opinions that are based on reason" (*Cambridge*, s.v. 'intelligence'), or "a very general mental capability that . . . reflects a broader and deeper capability for comprehending our surroundings" (Gottfredson 1997, 13), nor is it a cognitive process or even "a set of cognitive processes" (Cianciolo et al. 2004, 8). For example, plants express a Way of Being that nonconsciously and noncognitively informs how they are contextually with their environment (e.g., *Secret Life*, Tompkins 1973; *Brilliant Green*, Mancuso 2015; "Plant Cognition," Parise 2020).

Intelligence isn't cognition and doesn't imply consciousness or sentience–sapience. It transcends cognition which is not process-compartmentable anyhow but, like everything else in All Existence, is wholistic and holistic. Each aspect of cognition that one might call a cognitive process is wholistically integrated, interrelated, interdependent, and so on. Intelligence and cognition—"the use of conscious mental processes" (*Cambridge*, s.v. 'cognition') or "a variety of mental processes that allow us to maintain, understand and use information to create knowledge and reflect" (Dumper et al. 2019, par. 5)—are different things entirely. Though it's common to do so, conflating cognition with intelligence is inaccurate. Instead, intelligence expresses as cognition with respect to brain modality, as awareness with respect to mind modality, and as *unawareness* with respect to *unmind* modality.

In *The Story of Life*, the concept of unmind is plantlike. This means it noncognitively perceives relevant environmental reality, qualifies it with respect to own-self Way of Being in the context of the totality of environmental Way of Being, and applies a responsive, or regulatory, course of action. It isn't thinking; it's unaware. Science would say its awareness of and response to environment is mere biochemistry. But, in truth, it's more than that: it *is* Way of Being. Unmind intelligence is distributed awareness

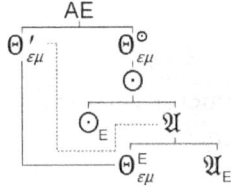

Fig. 2.1. Consciousness in context. The symbols in the image are as follows: AE is All Existence; $\Theta'_{\varepsilon\mu}$ is Energent–prime; $\Theta^{\odot}_{\varepsilon\mu}$ is Energent proto-life; $\odot$ is consciousness ($\mathcal{L}$ife); $\odot_E$ is totality of consciousnesses; $\mathfrak{A}$ is totality of universes; $\Theta^{E}_{\varepsilon\mu}$ is totality of universe Energents; $\mathfrak{A}_E$ is totality of existents within totality of universes. Dotted line indicates $\mathfrak{A}$ materially instantiates from Intentional instantiation by human consciousness embodying $\Theta'_{\varepsilon\mu}$.

whereas mind intelligence is unpropagated awareness, meaning it's wholistic. Unmind isn't consciously aware and doesn't experience cognition, thus we call its nonconscious awareness unmind (*SOL* § 2.2.1.1.2.1:237; *SOL* Table 5:235).

Cognition is simply one expression of intelligence where the modality is conscious–cognitive or nonconscious–noncognitive. Cognitive processes need not be as traditionally defined nor even conscious to be cognition. For more details on Way of Being, see CH. 2 § 6:86 and *SOL* § 2.2.1.1:234.

1.1.4 The Principal Aspects of All Existence

There are two principal aspects to All Existence: humanity, and everything else. Humanity emergently births 'in' Energent proto-life, a term for *Life-precursor proto-energy* that's an emergent property of Energent–prime, the fundamental 'energy,' or motivating force, of All Existence and therefore of our universe. Accordingly, Current All Existence—the fundamental reality in which we exist—comprises All Existence, Energent–prime, $\mathcal{L}$ife (in the literature, life is generally considered consciousness to varying degrees), and all universes along with their nonhuman life that humans build (*Fig. 2.1*). This is 'all there infinitely is.'

1.2 Your Mind

As noted, you are not your body. You are mind. Your mind is an aspect of your overall *personness*, which is Ḣuman and humanness ('Ḣuman' is humanity in every collective sense). You are emergently self-aware and altogether $\mathcal{L}$ife. Its functions of freedom, existence, choice, awareness, cognition, phenomenal awareness, qualia, and such are properties of the person, not of physical existence nor the body.

You aren't created by some deity. You are an emergent being because you emergently *birthed*. Your physical conception triggered your emergent birth as a self-aware proto-energy ℘erson. The term '℘erson' means the totality that is mind where mind is an emergent property of the self-aware proto-energy self. It differs from lowercase-p person used in the traditional sense. ℘erson defines ℒife; thus, ℒife *is* ℘erson. Thinkers traditionally distinguish two functional states of the person: awareness and existence. Each of these comprise their own many subfunctions. The former is loosely defined as consciousness and the latter as beingness, which in *The Story of ℒife* is personness. These functionalities of self-existent ℒife wholistically constitute consciousness and personness. Without such wholism, each aspect separately is merely (nonhuman) 𝕃iving, not ℒife—not ℌuman. A nonhuman entity that's alive is a 𝕃iving entity that thinks, feels, comprehends, and translates at whatever its capacity, including the human body sans ℒife mind. 𝕃iving is what we call 'alive' absent having ℒife. Matter comprises all 𝕃ivingness.

There are two fundamental 'energies' of All Existence. The first is emergent non-self-aware proto-energy. This is what we call Energent–prime in the context of All Existence and the Energent in the context of our universe. The second is self-aware proto-energy, which is ℌuman—in other words, you. When we use terms like ℘erson, ℌuman, self-aware proto-energy, ℒife, personness, humanness, and the like we are pointedly distinguishing you from both animals and embodiment as a unique, eternal human person. ℒife is unique to All Existence. It is only ever ℌuman. All other life is nonhuman; 𝕃iving entities created by humans in the context of the universes they build. Keep this in mind as you absorb and assess this chapter.

1.3 Embodiment

When your parents conceived you, what actually happened is that they conceived your body not *you*, the person. The process of conception *triggered* the start of your emergent birth 'in' Energent proto-life as a unique, non-duplicable entity—a ℘erson—which, in the process of mitosis leading from two cells to four in the zygote-cum-embryo, integrated your physical body. We'll cover this in CH. 2 § 2.3:49. For now, imagine the process of physical procreation as fertilization which then triggers your emergent birth that simultaneously integrates your embryonic body.

Physical embodiment is how you experience so-called phenomenal reality (SOL § 1:561). But recognize that you are not your embodiment. You are 𝕋hought, meaning thinking–feeling. You are also the mind in which it arises as well as the unembodied self that gives rise to mind that is the emergent self-aware proto-energy ℒife self—the very *you* that's you. Each ℘erson is emergently, autonomously unique and as infinite as All Existence. *This is what you fundamentally are.* What you're *not* is mere embodiment having dimensionality whether it's physical or spirit. The ℘erson who is aware of the reality of their existence flits amongst All Existence as easily as changing awareness from one venue to another, like working from home on a video call where your awareness flaps back and forth between children and colleagues. And in the spirit versus physical case, you manifest a spirit body anywhere your awareness is to experience that environment (SOL § 2.1.5.4:316).

You now have a generic understanding of All Existence as 'all there infinitely is' and yourself as mind transcendent of body. Let's flesh it out by delving into the origin of your body. This naturally includes the origin of humanity. The very first humans. Ever.

SECTION 2
Origin of the Body

The human person is an emergent self-aware being. You are a physical-born person because you were conceived by physically alive parents in the physical world. The physical-born most immediately live in the physical environment of our universe, although this is only one aspect of its larger construct. It's your physical existence that we now focus our attention on.

Recall from the previous section that All Existence is an emergent existent. Universes, however, though rooted in Energent–prime, are human constructs neither natural nor emergent. Prior to emergent ℒife, All Existence was nothing more than Energent–prime existing as existentiality but without reality, meaning absent human consciousness (SOL § 5:294). Then emergent ℒife entered the picture as an emergent existent of All Existence. Humanity developing awareness of All Existence transitioned it from mere existentiality to reality because *reality is only ever a property of human consciousness*. There is no such thing as reality absent human consciousness, which is to say, ℒife.

Humans then learned to build universes. When we think of 'all there infinitely is,' we can understand it overall as the environment of Energent–prime, emergent ℒife, and humanity's built universes such as our own. Those individuals who learned to embody Energent–prime *humanized* All Existence by Intentionally (CH. 6 § 2.1.1:143) building universes that are as infinite—indeterminate—as All Existence yet having time and space suitable for their phenomenal existents such as matter and nonhuman life as well as embodied humanity's phenomenal capabilities.

Humanizing All Existence means converting it from existing only as nondimensional, indeterminate—infinite *having no* time and space—existentiality having Way of Being to existing with a phenomenal—infinite *having* time and space—environment suited to all aspects of human reality (SOL CH. 20:301). Humanity, though an emergent existent of Energent–prime, 𝓛*ifeformed* All Existence to suit its own Way of Being. This is similar to physical life often terraforming—transforming—its immediate environment to suit its own Way of Being. 𝓛ifeforming All Existence through awareness of its Way of Being added dimensionality and determinance—time and space—and, accordingly, reality to All Existence. The first humans could have been satisfied to exist in their original unembodied, emergent proto-energy state and considered *that* existence to be all there was to be had. But such wasn't in their make-up, which is to say, their Way of Being; they're persons like us having the same curious thirst to explore, know, and experience.

When it comes to your human body recall that, in All Existence exclusive of human-built universes, there is only Energent–prime, Energent proto-life, and 𝓛ife where 𝓛ife is ℌuman. Accordingly, the only life is 𝓛ife. Its only form is ℌuman. This is 𝓛ife's Way of Being. 𝓛ife's environment naturally follows. Although we tend to think of nonhuman life—animal, insect, microorganisms—as 'alive,' this is life that humans created. We typeset it as lowercase 'life' in its traditional meaning and 𝕃iving in its wholistic sense (recall *The Story of 𝓛ife* typesets it as capital-L Living). Any emergent properties that arise in life over time—one such being random natural selection—originate in its human-Intentionalized Way of Being. Accordingly, life is 𝕃iving and not 𝓛ife, which is only ever emergently ℌuman. See the full discussion in SOL § 1.3:272.

Next, we describe humanity first arising in All Existence and then, along with you and me, how it came to be in our local universe.

2.1 Rise of the Humans

Most people are aware of monotheism's Adam and Eve story and science's take that modern humanity derives from a small, ancient, Stone Age population that evolved from a common ancestor connecting us with the apes. Even if these stories were true, they assume humanity exists nowhere else than Earth and that sentient–sapient life necessarily evolves local to its environment... thus, science fiction's plethora of crazy alien lifeforms as smart as (or smarter than) humans. But the absence of evidence is not evidence of absence and the assumption is incorrect.

Common belief justifies religious faith whereas common principles justify scientific faith. Philosophy with a capital-P is the traditional means by which these faiths seek to raise awareness of reality. Now there's a third way: energy testing as a common experience. Multiple individuals independently energy testing the same or similar answers to a given query falls in line with multiple scientific experiments justifying the same or similar conclusions to a given hypothesis. The story of humanity's birth that we tell below arises in validated energy testing. You can validate it yourself using your competent energy testing skill, should you choose to learn it. What follows is a summary of humanity's emergent birth long before our universe existed. You can read the larger story in *SOL* CH. 21:303.

2.1.1 Emergent Birth of the First Humans

It may sound mystically bizarre, science fictiony, or straight out of the radical quantum department to you, but our universe is one of many. This is because humans Intentionalize—build—universes. Altogether, these many universes constitute what *The Story of Life* never mind Marvel calls the *megaverse* (this isn't the *multiverse* theory that science ginned up). In the context of proto-energy, each universe is 'in' its own 'frequency space' that's of, and as indeterminate (infinite) as, All Existence.

As an analogy to help you visualize it, think of the megaverse as a radio dial and each universe a radio station frequency on that dial where All Existence is the entire electromagnetic radio spectrum. Alternatively, imagine All Existence like a megastore with the collective minds of all the shoppers within it as the megaverse where each individual shopper's mind is an individual universe. Take note, as well, of the distinction between *emergent existence*—Energent–prime, Energent proto-life, emergent *Life*—and *human-created existence* such as universes and the Living entities—animals, plants, microorganisms—that populate them which, en bloc, is All Existence. *Megaversal humanity* is all persons in all universes. *Universal humanity* is all persons in our universe, the very one you're living in right here.

Now, set that aside a moment. Let's go back to before any universe existed. Before any self-aware being existed. To when there was naught but All Existence *as* Way of Being and Energent–prime proto-energy its only aspect. In that milieu, Energent proto-life emergently arose as a *Life*-precursor proto-energy, which we've described in general terms along with the way emergent ℒife continues to birth 'in' Energent proto-life through the Intentionality of coupled humans to conceive.

The first incidence of self-awareness—ℒife—'in' All Existence occurred about 800 billion years ago. Two discrete, *self-aware proto-energy beings* emergently birthed 'in' Energent proto-life. Two *humans* birthed in *pairwise kinship* from ℒife-precursor Energent proto-life. We call them the Twins although the term is nothing like physical twins.

The analogy here with pairwise archí as matter's fundamental, unitized building block is compelling and intriguing (the archí is the fundamental origin of matter as an ultra-'charged,' super 'dense,' self-contained embolus of 'energy' analogous to an air bubble in near-boiling water that doesn't pop; defined in CH. 2 § 3.3.2.1:66). The reason is that both archí and ℒife initially independently arise in pairwise configuration. The analogy is weak, meaning imperfect, because an archí dephases if it fails to pairwise bond with another archí within a certain timeframe (SOL § 2.3.1:115). ℒife does not dephase if it fails to pair. It can't reproduce, either, which essentially is the same outcome as for unpaired archí that can't 'reproduce'—transition to complex matter—without pairing. This pairwise aspect of Energent–prime's Way of Being reflects throughout All Existence since 'all there infinitely is' ultimately constitutes from proto-energy. The more we comprehend All Existence, the more we see the warp and woof of its fundamental threads evident throughout. While this archí–ℒife analogy is true of archí since it's every archí's modus operandi, it's true only of the first two humans serving as monadic ℒife but not of emergent ℒife after them, which constitutes megaversal humanity.

The process by which ℒife initially birthed was the same as for any emergent ℒife; you, for instance. Except it wasn't a couple's Intentionality that triggered Energent proto-life's emergently coalescent differentiation, self-organizing, and completion as described in CH. 2 § 2.3.2:53 and SOL § 1.2.1.1:248. Rather, it was Energent proto-life that *spontaneously*—emergently—coalesced, differentiated, and self-organized 'within' its ℒife-precursor proto-energy 'at a point,' or 'Energent proto-life-place,' that was conducive—ℒife-precursive—at that moment to the emergent event. What emerged was not some weakly emergent aspect of typical (non-aware) proto-energy such as a new iteration of All Existence or some aspect of it. Rather, it was proto-energy having *self-awareness*, which is ℒife. It was at this point that first human ℒife *birthed*.

The Story of ℒife discourages using terms like 'emerged,' 'arose,' 'came into being,' 'instantiated,' and whatnot because we're talking 𝔥uman; ℒife, not non-*Life* (*Living*). It seems strange, perhaps, to think of our beingness this way. But recall that *Life* first births 'in' Energent proto-life as a transcendent, eternal *person*. When one conceives in a physically embodied state, it's only after emergent birth that one's body and mind sufficiently mature for their environment that the physical body births in the traditional sense out of their physical mother's womb. Accordingly, archetypal *Human* first birthed 'in' Energent proto-life in the same way that you, me, and the dogcatcher do as separate and distinct from embodiment.

In the seminal birth we're talking about here it wasn't a single birth, a single *Life*. Unlike biblical Adam from whose rib God later made Eve— Gen. 2:7, 21–22; incidentally, forming the primal theological-cum-cultural justification for woman's subordination to man that, as a fundamental human reality, doesn't exist—*two persons independently and simultaneously birthed* 'in' Energent proto-life. Each was a distinct, discrete emergent *Life*; altogether, pairwise humans. Twins.

A coin metaphor serves here. The coin is humanity and its geminous faces the Twins. Which one is the front or back doesn't matter; their births were simultaneous 'in' Energent proto-life (*see SOL* § 2:304 for a blow-by-blow account of first human emergence, the Twins discovering each other, and learning to use their minds). Although we reject astrology and the zodiac as fumes of fancy, we nevertheless represent our twin-faced coin with the handy Gemini sign (♊), because *Life*'s foundational Twins (vertical lines) established humanity (horizontal lines). In recognizing human emergence in the Twins, we discover *Life*'s primal, intrinsic equality of all persons as *emergent* beings, not *created* entities. This equality extends to male–female differentiation as well. Note, too, that the biological conventions of identical and fraternal twins don't apply at all to emergent *Life*. That's a reality only of physical embodiment.

2.1.1.1 Sex

Although each emergent *Life* is a person having unique Way of Being regarding personness, each person's Way of Being shares identity regarding humanness. This means each *Life* is indelibly *Human* despite being a unique *person*. Within this aspect of the person's Way of Being is a complemental differentiator vis-à-vis their personness that makes them, though the same *as* human, different. This complemental distinction *as* Way of Being is fundamental to embodied humans as it is with the Twins. Humanity calls it male and female according to body parts. Philosophy with a capital-P considers sex a person's fundamental reality: a male or female body means you *are male*, you *are female*. But humanity's main differentiator is not sexual organs with its attendant chemistry because ℒife emergently births *unembodied*. It therefore lacks all that. Neither is it childbearing assignment—sperm or egg—at conception, because that has no relevance outside the natural (physical) environment of a universe.

We can glean this truth from our spirit body, which lacks necessary metabolic chemistry or genetic childbearing assignment that defines or reflects sex. The reason is that in the supranatural (spirit) context *mind*, not *biology*, triggers procreation—emergent birth—regardless a male or female spirit body. Hence, *mind* defines sex, not body. Ideally, this is the case with physical embodiment, too, but not at present owing to The Corruption discussed on page 12.

The differentiation that we observe as the sexes lies in mindset as its expression and Way of Being as its fundament. Sex differentiation in our embodiment was initiated by the Twins, not by nature, evolution, or a deity. In this context, it's *generally* of a Way of Being *type* for each sex while subtly unique to the person. This is why ℒife birthed pairwise rather than a singleton. Because Energent proto-life's Way of Being itself is pairwise, emergent birth after the first two humans only triggers *with* pairwise ℒife—a couple—rather than with a singleton as it does with some 𝕃iving asexual, including same sex, reproduction. This is true even for unembodied humanity who live as mind without body (*sol* § 1.2.1:247).

This pairwise Way of Being differentiation that humanity calls sex is fundamental to ℒife therefore the Twins. But its embodiment as male–female archetypes in human culture roots in mindset, not ℌuman Way of Being and especially not in the body. An individual's encultured Way of Being embodies the *mindset type* of male or female. It's a chosen reality, not fundamental. Unembodied humanity sees this mindset-derived individual Way of Being in unmanifested—not embodied—pairwise terms whereas (physical or spirit) embodied humanity sees it manifested *as* their embodiment, *intrinsic to what they are*. Yet, it's only of the body and interchangeable anyhow. *Pairwise* differentiation is fundamental and (after the Twins' emergent birth) the only means to trigger emergent birth of ℒife. Male–female sex differentiation is habituated by, not fundamental to, the person. It's a mindset which early humans beginning with the Twins developed from our pairwise Way of Being that serves to express it in the context of embodiment (*sol* § 2.1.5:313).

The Twins are unique in this respect. They're humanity's firstborn who lived unembodied for a long time before building themselves integrable, physically procreative bodies (SOL § 2.1.5.5:322) that defined emergent pairwise differentiation as male and female. Being unembodied, they each birthed with this emergently unique aspect of Ꜧuman Way of Being which they discovered in themselves, and then embodied as a male–female archetype for procreation. Unlike their embodied progeny, they don't see themselves as male and female but as pairwise beings. Mina avers this distinction was forgotten amongst embodied humanity. For convenience, we call the Twins Mike and Molly. Maybe you prefer Molly and Mike, Thing One and Thing Two, or symbols like the "artist formerly known as Prince" (⚥). It makes no difference (cf. real names in SOL *Fig.* 145:337).

To recap, humanity doesn't differentiate as male and female simply premised on the physical body evolving sex in the natural environment. Instead, emergent ℒife's Way of Being that uniquely expressed in Mike and Molly's individual Ways of Being has, ever since, expressed *their* choice of sex to conceive physical-born, and subsequently spirit-born, children (SOL § 2.1.5.1:313). Our physical (and spirit) body's sex merely reflects ℒife's pairwise Way of Being. Those universe builders with whom we energy tested when writing *The Story of ℒife* consider it probable that the necessity of pairwise differentiation—sex—in Ꜧuman Way of Being came about in the first place simply as Energent proto-life's emergent tendency toward kinship such that 'no man should be an island' being, which is to say, the product of a singleton (SOL § 2.3.2.2:242). Their reasoning rests on our Way of Being's inability to be compelled arising pairwise with proto-love (*below*; SOL § 3.3.1:284), which makes for a Way of Being of uncompellable love. They observe that proto-energy itself operates in pairwise fashion across the spectrum whether with humans, archí, or even archí photons being pairwise with fundamental force.

Whatever its true genesis in the very first emergent birth of ℒife (the Twins), the pairwise nature of their emergence ensures that it takes two to tango with all the familial relations that naturally follow. Absolute freedom and absolutely two sexes—pairwise Ways of Being—trigger new emergent ℒife... you, for instance. That's humanity's wholistic Way of Being. We reference Mike and Molly as *he* and *she* according to their choice of sex. But *he* and *she* don't imply male and female so much as the pairwise aspect of Ꜧuman Way of Being in the context of triggering new emergent ℒife.

2.1.1.2 Proto-love

Proto-love is ℒife force the same way Intentionality is. The ordinary love we feel in everyday life emanates from proto-love, which is our *base dispo-*

sition. There's a reason human fetuses don't chow down on their womb mates like certain 𝕃iving creatures, and it's this fundamental, *emergently self-organized* disposition. It gives us an innate, intrinsic understanding of love—a pairwise expression—that inclines us ever to seek it.

Humans have such a rich tapestry of emotion because all feeling derives from the 'energy' of proto-love. Absent brain defects interfering with mind–brain integration, we spontaneously recognize and experience love. *The Story of ℒife* defines lowercase 'love' as its ordinary feeling and expression; all-caps 'LOVE' as the base emotion from which all (so-called negative or positive) feeling emotes; and 'proto-love' as ℒife force from which LOVE instantiates. Lowercase love is LOVE's *primary* expression (SOL Table 10:285). Proto-love isn't 'love' in any sense. It's simply *the* emotive force having a fundamental quality that humanity associates with the 'higher' (foundationally desired) aspects of human feeling. For a thorough discussion, see *The Story of ℒife* § 3.3.2:284.

2.1.2 The Meaning of ℌuman

Recall that Philosophy with a capital-P represents all types of inquiry as humanity's primary knowledge-seeking class of study. Yet, it's useful to recognize that the three principal modes of inquiry that we use to acquire data—empiricism, rationalism, revelation—and their principal subclasses of study from which we derive information—science, philosophy, theology—each interacts with and relies upon the others. Even so, they're hamstrung producing real knowledge of our natural and supranatural reality. There's no getting around it. It's counting sheep to reckon that next week or next year or next century their breakthroughs will render comatose our presently minuscule comprehension or majuscule suffering.

The tendency in science and philosophy to scorn the supranatural as unworthy of study and anyway in violation of their own sacred texts is simple bias. It follows from a lack of ready tools to collect data, the presumption no tools exist, and broadly accepted explanations based on the most obvious and accessible: physical nature. That's a myopic perspective at best, a hydra raising another head each time a new theory or observation posits the seemingly impossible or absurd. The real question is, what method can repeatably collect supranatural data that presents objectively and resolves to objective information, which veracity we can then repeatably establish? The answer is energy testing. In practice, it's revelation. So, the question is, how can revelation transition to data? This book isn't about energy testing, but you can catch a glimpse in CH. 9 § 3.1:192 or read SOL § 1.2:85 and SOL CH. 41:623.

With the above in mind, Philosophy with a capital-P's methodology to assess the nature and meaning of human traditionally subdivides into *consciousness* and *personness*. For it, consciousness is intellect–emotion, thinking–feeling, or awareness–self-awareness and personness is beingness, individuality, choice, uniqueness, or sanctity. This has borne no fruit whatsoever and not just from a lack of real data. It's because Philosophy with a capital-P is biased toward describing the what-is in terms of the how-is, which leads to conclusions that the what-it-does and the how-it-does-it must necessarily be the human reason for being and, hence, its what-is.

This reasoning underpins materialism, which is obvious, but spiritualism, too, which is less so. The reason is that for religion—theism and atheism alike—the human rationale embodies the seeming contradiction between two essential functionalities often erroneously interpreted from mind–body confusion as some aspect of dual beingness. The first aspect is the sacred tending toward spiritual awareness and higher instinct (morality) and feeling like love, worship of or attendance to a higher power or personified God, and so forth. The second is the profane tending toward physical awareness and lower instinct (base amorality–immorality) and feeling like hate, worship of or attendance to the observable world, and so on.

Religion's emphasis on these disparate functionalities that render us creatures of disparate natures, thus of disparate humanness—elevated on the one hand, debased on the other—mirrors materialism's own duality emphasizing our higher reasoning and baser instincts which leaves us in the same state. Each one's cure for the duality is functional—rooted in function—rather than humanness. Religion's lies in salvific rebirth and materialism's in evolutionary development.

The *person* is *Life*, a self-existing being of thinking, feeling, *translating*—motion, not rooted; no barriers to form, condition, nature—uniqueness, choice, and kinship. The first three terms typically reference consciousness, and the second three humanness. We categorize each set of three as *nature*, *way*, and *function* of existence. *Person* defines consciousness where *person* is *Human* (SOL Eq. 19.1:245). Thinkers traditionally distinguish two functional states of the person: awareness and existence. Each of these comprise their own many subfunctions. Awareness is loosely defined as consciousness and existence as beingness, which is personness. These functionalities of self-existent *Life* wholistically constitute consciousness and personness. Without such wholism, each aspect separately is 𝕃iving, not ℒife—not ℌuman. Since Philosophy with a capital-P generally wraps the ethereal notion of being—the person—in a functional veneer of consciousness, we parse that toward a fuller meaning of ℌuman in *The Story of ℒife* § 3.1:280. Here, we simply note the following.

Consciousness isn't definable as something with function, or a functional something. Rather, it's definable in its context, which is integration of humanness. The functionality that Philosophy with a capital-P traditionally ascribes to consciousness is properly the domain of ℒife. If we say, "Consciousness or the individual is this or that or has this or that functionality," then we're not properly referencing consciousness and personness but ℒife itself, because ℒife is ℌuman and ℌuman is ℒife. This means we can't properly explore consciousness and personness—its nature, function, existence, or any such thing—in the milieu typical of its inquiry by Philosophy with a capital-P. The reason is that it's acontextual of ℒife, the ultimate human context. If we divide consciousness and personness with rigorous distinction, we get each as functionality, meaning what each *does*, but not what each *is*. Therefore, we can't say what consciousness is—its what-is—because it doesn't have it. As an essentiality of ℌuman, consciousness is functionality in and of itself. So, consciousness without personness or personness without consciousness is 𝕃iving, not ℒife. 'Consciousness is personness' and vice versa means ℌuman, ergo ℒife: the indivisible what-is of consciousness and personness.

All that aside, we're human regardless how we look, act, think, or exhibit so-called human traits. This is because what makes us human aren't those attributes but simply ℒife, which is ℌuman. We *are* that ℒife; ergo, we *are* human in its Philosophy with a capital-P sense. It begins 'in' Energent proto-life but uniquely self-organizes *as* ℒife into a being *having* ℒife. Therefore, ℒife is human howsoever it manifests from one day to the next. Regardless how an individual rewrites his or her Way of Being into some vicious, hateful, sliming, acid spitting, giant purple people-eating disposition, he or she has ℒife; they're human. There are no such scary life forms having consciousness—having ℒife—in any universe. Persons whom you'd meet from another planet or universe are recognizably human howsoever unrecognizable they may appear in, say, culture and mindset. And that brings us to the human body.

2.2 Building the Human Body

You can read in *The Story of ℒife* the more comprehensive account of Mike and Molly discovering each other post-emergence, how Molly learns to create matter to build the first universe (the Primoverse), figures out the environment for their physical embodiment, then finally develops male–female sex (§ 2.1–2.1.5.1:305–313). In this section we focus on the creation of your human body and not the creation of *you*, who emergently births 'in' Energent proto-life in the process of your body's physical conception.

2.2.1 Evolution of the Human Body

Evolutionary theory inaccurately ascribes life and species development solely to *abiogenesis*—the natural process in which life arises spontaneously from non-Living matter—and random natural selection. Life instead arises and develops as a wholistic process involving all the environmental elements of our universe. The theory of evolution, as it's commonly understood, begins its analysis only with the functional end-state of biodevelopment. This isn't simply because the theory can't observe the mechanisms at work in chemogenesis, biogenesis, and mutagenesis (genesis of chemistry, biology, and that leading to mutation, respectively). It's because, until energy testing, no methodology could pry deeper to observe the unseen and formulate a means to empirically test it.

Science necessarily ends up viewing life as functionally nothing more than mystical chemistry. Yet, that's no less magical than claiming God did it. No matter how far from Darwin the modern, post-modern, and replacement syntheses get, they're only refining his thesis that life develops through a survival process that's effectively a natural (versus artificial, or, purposed) selectivity. These syntheses, originally coined by Julian Huxley in *Evolution* (1942) and then expounded by others, attempt to reconcile science's changing understanding of how life develops over time.

All living things except for mind–brain-integrated human bodies need to physically evolve. This means changing, altering, adjusting, or adapting. The reason is that, unlike supranatural matter, natural matter has independent existence, its own autonomous Way of Being. This organizes and operates its operational state in accord with the totality of its environment, which has its own Way of Being, too. Altering physical matter's Way of Being is an active process over time. For people as self-aware proto-energy, altering Way of Being is a *directed* affair. For nonhuman (Living) entities, including the human body absent mind–brain integration, altering—evolving—Way of Being is both *directed* and *undirected*.

2.2.1.1 Directed and Undirected Evolution

Evolution by random natural selection is only part of reality albeit for humans as persons versus their physical bodies it plays no part. Recall there are two fundamental aspects of living things: human ℒife and nonhuman 𝕃iving. In the natural environment, we distinguish between ℒife where mind–brain and mind–body integrates the 𝕃iving human body to form a wholistic, physicospirit embodiment and nonhuman 𝕃iving entities that make up the balance of all things we reckon as alive.

𝕃iving entities have Way of Being, and evolution occurs in two Way-of-Being contexts. First, when an imbalance between environment Way of Being and species Way of Being arises from environmental stressors, undirected Intentionality (SOL § 3.2:282) arises to rebalance these Ways of Being and *undirected evolution*—adaptive traits—may follow. Second, when Mina or other spirit persons directedly Intentionalize a change in an entity or species' Way of Being, then *directed evolution* may follow to the degree they coax along the change. Consequently, evolution of 𝕃iving entities is both an undirected and directed phenomenon. There are no stochastically unknowable factors behind evolutionary change. All change arises in specific contexts of which there are five that, to some degree, always overlap (Table 2-1). Further reading of this topic in *The Story of ℒife* pages 323–326 may be helpful.

2.2.2 Developing the Body's Form

Whatever material form Mike and Molly envisioned for themselves before Molly Intentionalized her universe—the Primoverse—now needed to comport with the realities demanded by its environment, itself the embodiment of Energent–prime's Way of Being. This means they had no control over how they could embody in her universe except regarding aesthetics (how embodiment *looks*, not *operates*; SOL § 2.1.5.3:315).

Without understanding reality as it is, humanity has believed the human body is the result of God's direct creation, random natural selection, or some faith-and-fact combo. Funnily enough, all three are at once correct and incorrect. There is no God in the traditional, deific sense, but a

Table 2-1: The five causes behind evolutionary change where matter–Energy means matter.

matter–Energy	Intentionality
Natural (undirected)	
Replication errors: chance occurrences	DNA internal
Emergent change	DNA internal
Environment pressure	DNA generally
Ultraculture	DNA generally
Artificial (directed)	
Human directed	DNA generally
Intentional directed (§ 6.5.2:437)	DNA generally

universe does have a founder—its builder—who develops physical human bodies in a way that comports with Ꜧuman Way of Being.

Our spirit bodies, however, are out of a builder's control. This is because it is ℒife itself that Intentionalizes—manifests—it at conception (SOL § 1.2.1.1.2:249). Thus, a builder can't evolve a physical human body different from what ℒife emergently manifests in the supranatural environment. The reason is that the self-aware proto-energy self—the *you* that's you— necessarily needs integrate a physical body matching the supranatural one, which is a direct manifestation of mind. The spirit body needs be a form that perfectly manifests Ꜧuman Way of Being, and this is what the emergent spirit body is: Ꜧuman Way of Being manifested. Accordingly, the physical body needs be the same form because *it must be mind-brain and mind-body integrable*. Otherwise, physicospirit integration fails and the 𝕃iving human body perishes.

The reality of our embodiment follows from ℒife's Way of Being and not a universe builder's whims because ℒife emergently births unique and autonomous (free). Thus, one can't alter emergent ℒife's Way of Being without its permission.

2.2.3 The Body Takes Shape

Molly built her universe, the first universe in All Existence, as a supranatural environment only. It had no physical environment like every subsequent universe because, at that point, the Twins had no inkling of a physical environment. That came later. Therefore, the first form of embodiment they developed was the supranatural body, the so-called spirit body. Note that the spirit body is all we're briefly describing in this and the following section to serve as a baseline for describing Mike and Molly later developing the physical body (SOL § 2.1.5.5:322).

The reason the supranatural environment thus the spirit body came first is easy to see. As a facsimile of proto-energy, supramatter's Way of Being is the Intentional reality of its builder (SOL § 7.1:212; recall that supramatter is spirit 'matter' as opposed to physical matter per CH. 1 PHYSICAL EMBODIMENT:6). It Intentionalizes—manifests, embodies—straight from Thought. It is, literally, manifested Thought. Matter in the natural environment has its own Way of Being that arises in the Energent of a universe, which is an aspect of Energent–prime, the fundamental proto-energy of emergent All Existence. Having an emergent origin rather than an Intentionalized origin, matter's Way of Being resists Intentional change. It's therefore more tedious to control whereas supramatter is neither resistant nor tedious. *Tedious* describes the nature of manipulating matter in its 'denser,' deterministic environment as more grueling; it's like forcing change on a powerful spinning gyroscope. For those unaware of Intentionality, tediousness demonstrates to them the impossibility of mind manipulating matter (SOL *Fig.* 94:218).

In contrast to the spirit body, the physical body needs develop by and through its physical environment. This takes time to accomplish since it only happens via directed evolution, which is Intentionality therefore tedious. While a physical body needs to function in its environment within certain parameters or not function at all, that's not the case with a spirit body having no objectively independent functionality of its own. The spirit body is a direct manifestation of Life's Way of Being. Mike and Molly created their first spirit bodies in terms of aesthetics based, in part, on what they thought they wanted to do with it. This included directly interacting with supramatter *as* supramatter to touch, move, and so forth. Later, they necessarily applied these spirit-body aesthetics to the physical body, adjusting its attributes over time as they developed it to meet the parameters necessary to survival in its physical environment as well as to integrate mind with body in the context of Human Way of Being.

As they experimented with physical form, they realized that Human Way of Being readily integrated certain ones over others. They couldn't, for example, Intentionalize a body with ten eyes, four arms, eight legs, two brains, and still *integrate* it; imagine the psychic break when dying as that physical body only to find yourself in a totally different spirit body. Such a dichotomized embodiment doesn't comport with Human Way of Being. With each effort to Intentionalize a form, it grew clearer that what emergently birthed 'in' Energent proto-life that we call 'Mike' and 'Molly' was a Way of Being gravitating toward a certain tangibility (supramatter) having a certain form and function. They had to narrow down what they'd initially imagined to a range of possibilities, eventually to specific attributes, then finally to an integration of attributes that altogether constituted a Way of Being-compliant embodiment in its totality. This is what we today call the human body. It is the only embodied Way of Being that integrates Human Way of Being.

In our ignorance of reality, it's been natural for us to think that God, evolution, or both created our body and only on Earth; that if there's intelligent life elsewhere in our universe then it necessarily has different, locally evolved bodies. In reality, the physicospirit body we have on Earth is more or less the same as on all inhabited planets in our universe. It's more or less the same physicospirit body that sentient–sapient life, which is necessarily Ꮒuman, has everywhere in all universes. Once the Twins figured out which form was Ꮒuman-Way-of-Being integrable, then *that was* our human form; the archetype. Down the line, they discovered their physical bodies could procreate emergent ℒife. Their emergently birthed physicospirit children then triggered the birth of new emergent ℒife habituating Mike and Molly's male–female pattern that further habituated down to us. Allowing for minor variation, it is habituated in us today. If you were to meet Mike and Molly in a physical or spirit embodied environment, their bodies would look essentially the same as your own.

Initially, Mike and Molly imagined two essentially identical spirit bodies compatible with Ꮒuman Way of Being but having no sex or procreative ability. This is because, having emergently birthed unembodied, they lacked any awareness they could even trigger the birth of new emergent ℒife. They thought the two of them was all there would ever be and planned accordingly. They manifested their spirit bodies via Intentionality with various attributes according to their own Ways of Being and personal preferences that fulfilled their principle desire to interact with each other by and through a *supramaterial* (spirit) environment. That task took about 100 thousand years to achieve. Their spirit bodies were supramaterial extensions of their mind in the spirit environment. They experienced their bodies in their supranatural reality.

As noted in Chapter 1 HOW THE PHYSICAL POWERS THE SPIRIT on page 18, the supranatural environment's energy comes from the natural environment. Hence, the natural Energent's proto-energy is necessary for spirit matter to endure. That being the case, their spirit bodies eventually required a physical universe to provide the necessary *enérgeia*. We use this Greek term in the sense of "the energetic essentiality of a thing's nature." It's the 'energy' that forms on the fly out of proto-energy in response to motion of matter. We define it in CH. 2 § 3.3.3.1:68. The natural Energent funding the supranatural Energent is the whole reason the physical universe and physical humanity even exists in the first place.

When Mike and Molly finally got around to working up physical life precursors circa 10 billion years later, the natural environment that Molly added to her universe took charge of developing all its complex structure based on her founding Intentionality for it. This is because the Twins didn't *engineer* the physical body or its environment. They simply Intentionalized its Way of Being. This is what guides the chemistry behind life precursors toward their Intentionalized end state until a physical human body, developed via directed evolution, is suitable for human integration. That task took about 20 billion years soup to nuts, from developing the precursors of life (SOL § 1.3.1:272) to arriving at an integrable physical body. This is double the approximately 10 billion years between our so-called Big Bang to Mina first initiating the general precursors to physical (Living) life, and the additional circa 3.5 billon years until he initiated the precursors for human embodiment on suitable planets. He started life precursors on Earth about 3.3 billion years ago (SOL § 1.1:532).

2.2.4 The Spirit Body Experience

The moment a spirit-embodied couple Intentionally conceives a child, a spirit body emergently manifests as part of Life's emergent birth 'in' Energent proto-life (SOL § 1.2.1.1:248). When a physical-embodied couple conceives where Intentionality *is* the fertilization process, a physical body biologically manifests in accord with its Way of Being. These dual embodiments of the self-aware proto-energy self mind–body integrate. This integrated, physical–spirit embodiment is physicospirit.

No one conceived Mike and Molly. They were a *spontaneous* emergent birth whereas all subsequent humans, like you and me, are a human-*triggered* emergent birth. Consequently, they emergently birthed 'in' Energent proto-life without integrating a body at all. Their lives began unembodied. Think of a sensory deprivation tank—a dark, soundproof tank filled with a foot or less of salt water, also called a float or isolation tank—as an analogy for the unembodied state before Mike and Molly discovered each other. Here, Thought was their only stimulus hence reality. Accordingly, they were free to manifest a spirit body and integrate a physical body at will since they were alone in All Existence (one can't integrate an already-integrated physical body, thus no one can freely integrate your body while you, being physically alive, integrate it; cf. SOL § 3.2:566; *see also*, SOL § 1.2.1.1.3:250; SOL § 2:564; SOL § 3.2.2:567).

After Molly created her universe, she and Mike manifested a spirit body long before the natural environment there could support a physical body. They weren't in a rush to create physical bodies anyhow as they didn't know it was necessary to a universe's spirit environment. Once they knew, the learning curve to formulate physical life was steep. Besides, they procrastinated. They knew nothing of any aspect of human existence until they experienced it . . . there was just so much to experience and learn with a spirit body! Even today, people encounter previously undiscovered human capabilities—breaking the four-minute mile; Intentionalized healing—and there is zero probability that'll ever cease. The human psyche integrating Energent proto-life thus interacting with Energent proto-energy is astoundingly rich, complex, deep, and broad. Your life according to this understanding of our human origin is breathtakingly vast.

Once the Twins comprehended Intentionality and Molly had built her Primoverse, manifesting a spirit body was pretty much a breeze. More difficult was exactly *what* to manifest. As described, only a body in accord with Ƕuman Way of Being integrates the human mind. Suppose the Twins Intentionalized a physical spider-like creature via directed evolution with which to integrate their mind. This effort would fail because the overall form is outside Ƕuman Way of Being; it couldn't evolve a brain that would integrate mind. Manifesting one's already existing spirit embodiment as a spider-like spirit creature is certainly doable because of Intentionality. Some spirit persons manifest all manner of forms for different occasions. But creating it to physically integrate a ℘erson is not. Accounting for these nuts and bolts took the Twins considerable time.

2.3 Birth of You and Your Body

ℒife isn't a biological emergent as aliveness is with 𝕃iving—nonhuman—entities (*SOL* § 1.3:272). It's not a function of our universe. Mina, who built our universe, didn't *design* it. He didn't *engineer* it. ℒife is independent even of All Existence. ℒife is its own existent. That's why properties, or functions, of ℒife such as self-awareness, choice, and freedom are intrinsic to human existence and not granted by an all-powerful deity, nature, government, religion, philosophy, ideology, or the individual to seize or dispense at will. Nor that 'created equal' means only equality in human creation—equality *of* persons *in* birth—and not equality in being, which is all forms of equality *between* persons *in* relationship and is both a choice and a freedom (*SOL* § 5.1:428; *SOL* CH. 36:585).

Earlier, we made a distinction between the Twins as a spontaneous emergent birth and all others a triggered emergent birth via pairwise humans. Emergence is nevertheless, by definition, spontaneous. Therefore, all human life *as* ℒife is spontaneously emergent. The difference is that no pairwise humans triggered Mike and Molly's emergent birth. It was *undirectedly* emergent. You, me, and all humanity besides the Twins are *directedly* emergent.

𝓛ife emergently births spontaneously 'in' Energent proto-life when the intention of pairwise persons to procreate becomes Intentionality. This simply means that one achieves a state of mind—not a mental state but one of personness, as it's your entire being involved and not simply the conscious content of your mind—that exerts an Intentional effect (in this context) with respect to Energent proto-life. It then responds to this Intentionality in coalescent differentiation 'at a point in' Energent proto-life where it's conducive—meaning a 𝓛ife-precursor—to the Intentionality until a *critical Intentionality threshold* obtains and 𝓛ife emergently births. What we've described here is only an approximation of what's happening, as we lack suitably conceptual language to fully describe it at this time (*SOL* § 2.3.2.2:242). Before moving on, let's describe Energent proto-life.

2.3.1 Energent Proto-life

Energent proto-life (EPL) is a 𝓛ife-precursor proto-energy that's an emergent property of Energent–prime proto-energy. Recall this latter 'energy' is the totality of All Existence, meaning 'all there infinitely is,' and includes our universe. Energent proto-life as a 𝓛ife-precursor proto-energy is an emergent property of All Existence. It's as indeterminate—infinite—and without time or space as All Existence and proto-energy, and suffuses All Existence thus our universe.

As an analogy to visualize this, think of All Existence as an ancient, primitive sea where Energent proto-life is the chemistry precursor to sea life that spontaneously—emergently—arises in that environment; science calls this *abiogenesis*. Naturally, Energent proto-life differs from Energent–prime's nonconscious proto-energy in the same way the chemistry precursor to sea life differs from the general chemistry of the inorganic material of the sea. Energent–prime's proto-energy and Energent proto-life are wholly distinct. They reside in unique 'frequency spaces' just as universes reside distinct from others and Energent–prime (and inorganic chemistry resides in the sea distinct from life's chemistry). Yet they are, altogether, All Existence (the sea). 𝓛ife emergently birthed in the context of Energent proto-life.

When we say that 𝓛ife as Mike and Molly is an emergent, we don't mean it sprang into existence from constituents. Rather, its emergence was a spontaneous eruption of self-awareness 'in' Energent proto-life. This is conceptually the same way that archí spontaneously erupt from our Energent as matter and is analogous to sea life spontaneously arising in the

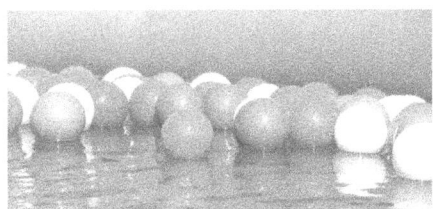 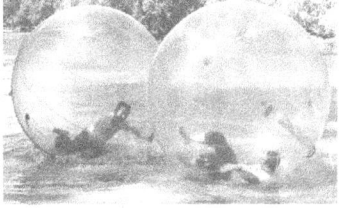

Fig. 2.2. Left, analogous schematic of instantiated (individual) 𝓛ife 'in' EPL 'solute' as EPL-discrete, dimensional 'balls' floating in a non-dimensional EPL 'sea.' Right, a thought experiment: people in balls represent discrete minds in touch via EPL 'water' with others and the whole universe and megaverse.[1]

context of life's chemistry precursors and not the inorganic chemistry of the sea. 𝓛ife as a being—not consciousness as an expression of 𝓛ife—is a kind of 'matter' in that, in the context of Energent proto-life, it is 'spatially' finite as a mode of existence (as an existent) yet nonspatial and indeterminate—infinite—as a mode of being (as a function; *Fig. 2.2*). In the context of our sea analogy, any individual sea life is spatially finite as an existent yet infinite as a function in that it can move, reproduce, and evolve.

With Energent proto-life, 'matter' doesn't mean something tangible or physical. It signifies in the Energent proto-life context an instantiation of 𝓛ife that differs in nature from Energent proto-life similar to how an amoeba differs from its chemistry precursors. This difference is what we're loosely calling a spatial, dimensional existent. While an individual 𝓛ife such as you is a discrete yet indeterminate being, it isn't discrete the way an archí is discrete, nor indeterminate the way Energent proto-life is indeterminate. In terms of our spatially oriented universe, 𝓛ife is determinate in 'space' and this is a valid corollary for nonspatially oriented Energent proto-life even though, as you can see, there's a substantive conceptual distinction.

Emergent 𝓛ife in and of itself isn't infinite the way our universe is—say, in terms of dimensional space. For example, your self-aware proto-energy self is not spatially infinite like outer space. It's 'discrete,' 'finite,' 'contained' the way an archí is even though the archí itself *is* encapsulated proto-energy without time or space. Yet, it *is* infinite in the sense that, suffused 'in' Energent proto-life, your consciousness can have awareness of any part of it and any reality thereby and interact with it. Essentially, a person *is* Energent proto-life—as infinite as All Existence though in and of itself not All Existence—who emergently birthed in that milieu as self-existence.

While 𝓛ife is entirely unrelated to matter, it relates to dimensionality. It exists in a discrete and dimensional state that's not directly translatable to how we spatially comprehend discrete and dimensional. We can think of it as 'Energent proto-life-discrete' and 'Energent proto-life-dimensional' as a way to conceptually demarcate Energent proto-life's reality from our own dimensional reality of space and time. This is the reason we use single quotes for spatial terms (e.g., 'in,' 'out of') when referencing Energent proto-life. Imagine going inside an archí: you'd transition from dimensionality having time and space to nondimensionality having no time and space.

Since consciousness interacts with all consciousnesses, a person (embodied or unembodied) can be aware of and interact with all humanity via Energent proto-life. Since Energent proto-life also suffuses therefore interacts with Energent–prime, a person can be as aware of, and Intentionally interactive with, the Energent of a universe and any entity of said universe as they can with Energent–prime overall. This is the foundation of Intentionality. Energent proto-life is proto-energy just as Energent–prime is proto-energy and the natural Energent of a universe is proto-energy. ℒife force energizes 'in' and emergently emanates 'from' Energent proto-life. This is ℒife.

Mike and Molly, the first two humans to emergently birth, were a spontaneous emergence 'in' Energent proto-life as novel life. Each was unique, aware, and self-aware. Since then, humans conceive—trigger emergent birth of—humans via pairwise Intentionality. Thus, conceived ℒife emergently births 'in' Energent proto-life just as Mike and Molly did except not spontaneously but *Intentionally*. Two persons (your parents, for instance) conceive—Intentionalize—a new ℘erson. Their Intentionality—fertilization—stimulates a nascent emergence 'in' Energent proto-life which coalescently differentiates and self-organizes into novel ℒife; in this case a unique, individual person: *you*.

Novel emergence is why each person is unique and absolutely autonomous. ℒife can never be duplicated. Ever. The thinking of such universe builders as Mina on why no more and no less than two pairwise persons can conceive is because emergent ℒife arose in a societal context as a kinship pair, not singular or as a group. This is pairwise in the ℌuman context. Hence, the conditions of emergent procreation itself also emergently arose as a kinship experience. This is the reason humanity's Way of Being is intrinsically familial, rooted in proto-love. Both are aspects of ℌuman Way of Being intrinsic of Energent proto-life.

Energent proto-life is the 'medium' that allows a consciousness to interact with others and with proto-energy beyond so-called normal means. As a ℒife-precursor proto-energy, Energent proto-life is distinct from nonconscious proto-energy, which is Energent–prime or a universe's Energent. It resides as a different expression to Energent–prime that's weakly analogous to the way the natural and supranatural environments are different expressions of our universe's dual-purpose (spirit–physical) yet still singular Energent. Put differently, Energent–prime and Energent proto-life discretely exist in All Existence as separate yet relational, noncontiguous yet interactive proto-energy entities.

Consciousnesses communicate or interact with each other and all of the All Existence environments through both Energent–prime proto-energy and Energent proto-life in exactly the conceptual way that all 𝕃iving and ℒife entities of a universe communicate or interact via their own universe's Energent (e.g., quantum 'entanglement' in the ℒife and 𝕃iving contexts).

2.3.2 Emergent Birth of ℒife

Procreative Intentionality as it *currently* operates in our physical environment comes in two forms: 'energy' of mind and 'energy' of biology. Our conscious or subconscious intent produces mind Intentionality. With physical procreation, Intentionality lies in the biology itself, sperm being a biological Intentionality in its own right. This means it constitutes out of biology's ineluctable process without need of mind Intentionality at all, although Intentionality does affect the conception.

For example, whereas unintended procreation is a bane of physical sex because the biological process of fertilization operates in our current context regardless intent, it doesn't occur with spirit procreation unless a pairwise couple Intentionalizes it the same way in all respects (*SOL* § 1.2.1.1.2:249). Here's how emergent birth of ℒife happens in the physical context.

Physical procreation working through cell division undergoes a series of checkpointed—interruptible—biologically Intentionalized operations in three phases (Hartwell 1989, 630; Hunt et al. 2011, 3495). Checkpoints are control mechanisms—potential termination points—in the cell cycle that ensure proper cell progression. There are three main checkpoints but only two of them, the G_2/M and the anaphase–telophase (spindle) checkpoints, are relevant to emergent ℒife. These two checkpoints ensure there's no cell replication until biology repairs problematic DNA and that duplicated chromosomes don't separate until properly attached to the cell's cytoskeletal structure (spindle), respectively.

The events happening within these two checkpoint periods provoke birth of ℒife over three phases that *The Story of ℒife* terms *coalescent differentiation*, *self-organizing*, and *completion*. However, if for whatever reason in this methodology the cell division process goes out of spec at any one checkpoint, then cell division stalls for repair or fails. In the latter case, the biology ceases production (e.g., Green 2014, 1466c). Each checkpoint in the physically procreated birth of emergent ℒife is as follows (*see* the full discussion in *SOL* § 1.2.1.1.1:248).

2.3.2.1 Birth of ℒife: Phase One

Emergence of ℒife begins with a *coalescent differentiation* of Energent proto-life. It's a reaction to the biological creation of a unique, self-existent being in the context of two self-aware proto-energy individuals.

Energent proto-life (EPL) triggers in physical procreation. During mitotic cell division following sperm–egg fertilization whereby a cell divides in the cleavage subprocess toward developing into an embryo, the internal parts of a fertilized cell's single-nucleus (the zygote) first gather up the nerve to separate over the course of the (early and late) prophase and metaphase stages of *mitosis*. This is the cellular process where replicated chromosomes separate into two new nuclei.

2.3.2.2 Birth of ℒife: Phase Two

The emergent ℒife process 'in' EPL then moves into *self-organizing* when the zygote successfully divides its single nucleus into two nuclei—this while still a single cell where actual cell division hasn't yet initiated—over the course of the anaphase and about 70% of the telophase (prior to cytokinesis) stages. The developing person (let's say it's you) has nascent ℒife at this point but not humanness—it embodies none of ℌuman Way of Being—until this first cell division from single nucleus to two nuclei successfully completes (ibid Hartwell, Green).

During this phase, there's feedback from the 'energy' of biology to Energent proto-life where biology–EPL establishes co-awareness. If cell division goes out of spec, EPL response ends and there's no emergence of ℒife, therefore no physical conception; think of a tornado building only to dissipate before achieving sustainable rotation. This feedback happens because EPL, having no time and space, suffuses not just Energent–prime but every speck of our universe including the fertilized cell. But, as with ℒife, it's a *vitae mysterium*, too. Universe builders understand *how* the process works—the developing emergent being 'in' Energent proto-life only continues if it's getting in-spec feedback from the 'energy' of biology—but not *why* the *phenomenon* works. It's the mystery of ℒife.

Following successful first-cell division—two discrete cells now comprising the zygote-cum-embryo—but before these two cells begin their internal mitotic process leading to next cell division (from two cells to four), biology–EPL co-awareness conveys to Energent proto-life that the biology is a stable, in-spec creation. This feedback process, intrinsic of proto-energy as well as of Energent proto-life, is how Mina knew within a picosecond—a trillionth, or 1×10^{-12}, of a second—that our universe was in spec and operating and developing as intended. That his Intentional contribution to creation was over. That the universe would self-develop from that point in accord with its Intentionalized Way of Being. *The Story of Life* terms the cell division process in this second phase *first mitosis*.

2.3.2.3 Birth of Life: Phase Three

Finally, the continuation of biology's in-spec feedback to Energent proto-life permits the nascently emergent being to finish self-organizing and move to *completion*. In this phase, the coalescently differentiated and self-organized nascent Life at the EPL *creational focal point*—this is the 'point in' Energent proto-life conducive, i.e., Life-precursive, at that very moment to the birth of emergent Life (coterminous with your zygote's spatial location)—reaches the critical Intentionality threshold. This is the moment before which there wasn't and after which there is an eternal, self-existent human person having Life: *you*. This occurs immediately upon about 50% of *second mitosis*, meaning two internally divided cells moving toward four separate cells, which completes it. Now, each of these cells completes second mitosis. This phase begins and ends with the same mitotic stages as phases one and two (Hartwell, Green).

Perhaps a helpful way to visualize the process of emergent birth 'in' Energent proto-life is to imagine the energy you'd see in a science fiction movie coalescing until it was visible, becoming more defined and dense until ending, say, as a 'ball of light' that's a newly existing entity—in this case, a self-aware human person. Then, imagine this sci-fi energy automatically integrating—entangling—the above-described clump of cells in the womb that, altogether, grows into and then births as a physical-born, Human-integrated physicospirit baby.

2.3.3 Birth of Your Physicospirit Body

In an ideal world not subject to the vagaries of gestation, correct human body development is inevitable from Phase Three. Unfortunately, we don't live in an ideal world but one in which things go wrong between embryo and birth. So, it's important to understand that the Way of Being of Energent proto-life is a singular stimulus-response to procreation initially mediated to some degree in the physical case by its awareness of the 'energy' of biology. Bear firmly in mind that Energent proto-life does not create bodies but births 𝓛ife. Bodily procreation is simply the agent provocateur to Energent proto-life's creational Way of Being the same way a doctor's mallet to your knee provokes, or stimulates, your body's reflexive Way of Being. The biological process proceeds as an automaton that self-creates in accord with its Way of Being subject to any biological errata that don't self-correct for reasons discussed later in this book.

One can readily surmise that phase three completion means a self-existent human being—you—emergently births regardless subsequent biological cessation (death) at any point forward. This has implications for abortion and cloning used to harvest human stem cells (primarily somatic cell nuclear transfer; SOL § 2.2:410). Both of these terminate a body's development after second mitosis, which is *after* 𝓛ife's emergent birth. This causes a developing 𝓛ife to be abandoned by albeit not separated from its physical body and it goes into stasis. Though still nascently self-aware, its further development into mind consciousness halts without a spirit person's hands-on intervention. This in turn halts further *spirit body* development, too. However, we note a happy caveat.

In November 2021, Mina surprised us with news that, consequent to post-Big Healing changes (TBH, SOL CH. 4), one particular physicospirit person's 𝓛ife force had saturated our universe similar to how Mina's own does. As a consequence, unfound or ignored aborted or prenatally dead persons' 𝓛ife selves had been coming out of stasis since July 12, 2020, their spirit bodies 'waking up' to resume development. Even without hands-on human intervention—spirit persons integrating 𝓛ife force via direct care—these fetuses resumed mind–spirit-body growth and development toward adulthood they would've otherwise had in the womb. This marked the first seminal change in physicospirit life since the Big Healing (SOL § 2.2.2:412).

2.3.4 Conclusion to Origin of the Body

You now have a generalized concept of how Mike and Molly initiated physical life to occur in the natural environment of Molly's Primoverse, from its initial terrestrial life precursors to a human body integrable with 𝓛ife and all its capabilities. Mina followed the same process to establish physical life and human embodiment in our universe.

Now, in order to understand how your body actually exists and operates in this world toward an understanding of Intentional healing and why it works, we first need a basic comprehension of our universe and the 'energy' that supports it and therefore your body.

Section 3
The Milieu in Which Your Body Lives

The notion you're an eternal person with a physical body that infinitely responds, healthwise, to your eternal mind has implications needing a discussion on the universe in which you find yourself and the energies that power it and, accordingly, your physical body. The reason is twofold.

First, our universe is Mina's Intentional creation, a product of his mind, of Thought. It's therefore an aspect *albeit not in nor a part of* Mina's mind. It's a separately manifested aspect of All Existence; a distinct, independent existence therefore reality. His mind, as with every human mind, is *infinite* and *eternal*, which are terms for *space indeterminate* and *time indeterminate*. Second, the 'energies' of our universe are the 'energies' which you manipulate with your mind to manifest physical healing.

This section clarifies the 'energy' that suffuses every aspect of your existence, and that your mind is not limited to your brain. Some of it's a bit technical, but don't let that discourage you if that's not your thing. It isn't necessary that you master this information for you or a healer to heal your body. But if you want to heal *everything* in your own body yourself without a healer, then the information in this section is necessary because you need to understand 'energy' for that. If that side of science interests you then read SOL CH. 17:111 for a seriously full dose of this section's rather deboned discussion. Either way, let your subconscious absorb what follows. And enjoy the journey.

3.1 Space Infinity

What are we to say about infinite space? We all live within it here on planet Earth. Unlike intangible time, with space we're talking about a seeming existent, something real and tangible . . . and yet, we're not. Sure, we can fly spaceships through it. See light traverse it. Experience its near vacuum. Find all things there. We exist in its context. Yet, like infinity and time (SOL CH. 14:93; SOL CH. 16:105), the apparent boundless extent that is space isn't a *thing*, either. Accordingly, it can't be infinite in the way we typically think of a thing as infinite—as some sort of a completed whole, an infinite set of matter, an endless space, or the like. The norm is to see space as a physical reality that has expanse. That's why we think of its infiniteness dimensionally as endless volume, size, or distance. This dimensionality is why some believe the very concept of infinity, thus eternity, is impossible and human life is therefore materialistic and finite.

Although indeed it's a physical reality, space only has *expanse*—a relational term for a definable scope between referents, as something has expanse only in context—in the presence of relational, detectable objects from galaxies to dust to gas. In short, *matter* (SOL § 2:114). Beyond where there are detectable objects, there is no expanse. Space has expanse between our Milky Way galaxy and the Andromeda galaxy, for instance, because there's a measurable relationship between these observable galaxies that provides context for it. That expanse is approximately 2.54 million light-years in terms of the distance product of velocity and time ($d=vt$). If we flew a spaceship from one to the other, we could measure our passage and the expanse using one or both galaxies as referents. But what's the expanse of space beyond its farthest object, beyond even its light?

Science generally postulates a universe that's infinite in expanse, size, or volume. For example, scientists calculate the average number of subatomic particles in a cubic chunk of the observed universe on the basis that there are finite configurations for these particles (e.g., quarks, leptons). Scientists feel that if there are infinite particles in an infinite universe (or maybe the multiverse, which is *not* the aforementioned and entirely different megaverse), there must be infinite quantum outcomes for these particles. Therefore, these finite configurations must repeat at some point. Not only that, but the configurations of particles that are *you* must also repeat because science sees you as nothing but matter. Thus, in the 'many worlds' and other multiverse theories, there are infinite numbers of sentient–sapient you living different lives with different outcomes. Because . . . infinity.

However, while elementary particles or even molecular configurations do have finite possibilities, archí configurations are infinite. A body, for example, is configured from molecules that constitute from atoms that constitute from subatomic structures all built up from single, bonded-archí pairs. At the molecular or atomic level, it seems to science that a body must be configurably finite therefore duplicable in an infinite universe. But underlying seemingly identical subatomic particles such as leptons, quarks, or bosons are configurably differing—infinite—archí configurations. The reason is that archí substructures are in constant flux because of Energent 'undulations' (Eq. 17.95 in SOL § 6.11.2:194). Archí substructure 'energies' are what ultimately lie behind matter forming into specific macrostructures like atoms, Earth, or your body at any specific moment. As those 'energies' are always in flux then, even with identical molecules, it's impossible to form identical macrostructures. Therefore, with the current scientific awareness of reality, there's no reason to presume duplicate matter—another Earth, another you, another ham sandwich with an ounce of mayonnaise on it—will or even could occur. It's an irrational assumption.

From science's vantage, the luminous, normal matter—what interacts electromagnetically and gravitationally with other matter and radiation—that it detects as the observable universe could be all there actually is. In this case, if space has infinite expanse then, beyond the farthest objects (not counting elementary and composite subatomic particles), it would be object-less and therefore expanse-less. If you flew a spaceship at lightspeed c for infinite time in that context, you'd never encounter a physical end to space, to be sure. More to the point, you'd be in a measureless void, unable even to know if you were, in fact, moving. In such an expanse-less environment, what then would infinite space in actuality be?

3.2 Fundamental Energent

Well, indeed, that's how our universe came into being in accord with Mina's Intentionalized Way of Being for it. All material existence in the form of atomic objects are concentrated right here where we detect them because this is the locality, called the observable universe within our infinite universe, where human consciousness physically embodies (SOL § 4:150). Beyond the observable universe (not all of which we can presently observe) is object-less space, and this reality has implications for the very concept of infinity (SOL CH. 14:93). It's not entirely empty space, of course. Besides subatomics, there's what *The Story of Life* calls the *Fundamental Energent* (or, simply, *Energent*). It's a universal permeant that's the root source of existence in our universe. Mina calls what expresses from it *real energy* (though not as a property of the Energent) as opposed to *force*, or *applied energy*. It is, to cite Mina, "*the* fundamental resource agency and instrument of power and energy in our universe."

Energent–prime, being of All Existence, suffuses every aspect of All Existence. This naturally includes our universe, where it 'flows' into the natural (physical) environment of our local Energent like an ocean into a bay as a function of the process of Intentional creation (SOL § 6.10:186). In the context of our universe, it's the *Energent*. Thus, the Energent of our universe *is* Energent–prime. When we mention one, we necessarily reference the other. We distinguish between them, however, according to whether a discussion is focused on All Existence or on our universe.

Energent–prime can only be described *as* Way of Being. It's an *expression* of proto-energy, the fundamental 'energy' of All Existence as above, and is *of* 'energy' but not 'energy' itself. Proto-energy is not 'energy' in any way that scientific much less spiritualist thinkers imagine it. This is why we typeset 'energy' in single quotes. It's similar to the way that All Existence ('all there infinitely is') isn't a thing, an existent, or even a reality but simply Way of Being.

Mina doesn't describe Energent–prime *as* Way of Being the way he describes All Existence although it *has* Way of Being. He describes the Energent *as* Energent–prime being the motivating 'energy' of our universe in just the same way that Energent–prime is the motivating 'energy' of All Existence. Besides typesetting 'energy' in single quotes as a visual aid to distinguish it from any other concept of energy you may have, we also use single quotes when referencing traditional understandings of energy like 'waveform,' 'wavelength,' 'density,' and many others in the context of the Energent versus in the context of physical universe matter and its fundamental energies that science observes.

By way of analogy, imagine the Energent as (altogether) the energies in the ocean that makes water do what it does—say, from wind, temperature, and oxygenation to motion, weight, and tides. Science can observe these physical energies because they're force, meaning applied energy it can measure. But it's the 'energy' of the Energent that's behind nature's fundamental force such as the electromagnetic or strong and weak nuclear forces that give rise to these physical forces. Because of this, we call the 'energy' of Energent–prime *proto-energy* because it's the *Intentional* origin of our universe and the (weak) *emergent* origin of matter and all its energies. In other words, proto-energy is an *emergent property* of All Existence notwithstanding All Existence as an expression of proto-energy.

Proto-energy is proto 'energy' similar to how a proto-human is the proto body of the integrated human. Unlike with invisible 'energies' (*vs.* the applied energies science can observe and measure) in the context of the ocean, we necessarily need a different kind of science to observe and measure proto-energy. We call it *Energent science* and *Energent physics*.

3.2.1 The Energent of Our Universe

In and of itself, the Energent is without traditional waveform by which science observes and measures the applied energies of our universe with which you're most familiar. It's infinitely just there. Ever in 'motion.' Brought into being *as* our universe by Mina not magically, divinely, or in some fantastical way but with Intentionality, which we describe in detail in Chapter 6 and *The Story of Life*. Six descriptors define the Energent for our purposes here. It's the:

> 1) binding force of the universe; 2) lowercase-l life (i.e., Living) 'energy' of the universe; 3) supranatural (spirit) 'energy' source; 4) medium through which all things interact and have awareness of each other; 5) medium through which Mina interacts—loosely described in THE BIG EVENT as 'quantum entanglement' (TBH § 1.5:34; SOL § 1.5:16)—with the totality of the universe; and 6) expression of the primary Energent, i.e., Energent–prime, of All Existence.

It underlies the fundamental forces of nature, there being eight, not four, in total (gravity isn't included, as it's a fundamental force *phenomenon*; SOL § 3:119). These are:

> 1) Archí Force AF, 2) Strong Nuclear Force SNF, or strong interaction; 3) Weak Nuclear Force WNF, or weak interaction; 4) Electromagnetic Force EMF; 5) Parity Force PF; (SOL § 6.11:191); 6) Field Force FEF (note: typeset as Ff in SOL); 7) Métier Force MF; and 8) Flavor–color Force FCF. See SOL § 1:112.

In the natural environment of our universe, the Energent is invisible but detectable, exerting its presence throughout. We sometimes experience it as unexplained heat in our body—mainly the spine, a sort-of 'antenna'—when intensely emoting or bringing it into the body for healing. There's a supranatural Energent, too. Aware persons can manifest it (and the natural one) in such a way as to perceive it as something like a hazy heat wave. The supranatural Energent depends for its existence on the natural Energent because the former is Mina's Intentional creation (*below*).

The Energent's 'energy' harkens back to the start of our universe, the first 10^{-43} second that's called the Planck epoch. As an expression of Energent–prime, it's the 'energy' of creation itself. As noted in Chapter 1 and above, it originates in the equivalent Energent–prime of All Existence that transcends our universe with which Mina Intentionally brought our infinite universe into being . . . you didn't think it popped out of nowhere in some big bang, did you?

The Energent permeated our infinite universe since the get-go, as it's really just Energent–prime in the context of our universe. It empowers everything natural and supranatural in our universe to exist and operate. It is, in some ways, analogous to fundamental force (as the physical expression of the Energent) empowering everything physical to exist and operate in the ocean, on the planet, in the solar system and galaxy, and throughout the observable and the infinite universe.

Although the natural and supranatural Energents of our universe are discrete, the former's 'energy' translates to the latter's in a synergic relationship because only physical processes manufacture it. The natural environment powers the supranatural one, as the latter makes no 'energy' of its own. Instead, 'energy'-producing physical processes continually harvest the natural Energent and translate that 'energy' to its supranatural twin, a net 'energy' consumer. The natural Energent where we physically live is a net producer although, from the perspective of All Existence, our universe itself is a net 'energy' consumer whereas All Existence is a net producer. In short, the natural environment is the power plant for the supranatural one, where a bit over three-quarters of humanity in our universe lives.

To recap, the Energent comprises a proto-energy from which fundamental force energizes and emanates. It's not *applied* energy in the sense that people scientifically and popularly cognize the concept of energy as work or force. It's quintessentially more an *élan vital* (life force) in that it indelibly enlivens the system from its initial, full entropy microstate of zero 'energy' to its one and only possible hence irreversibly ensuant dynamical, zero entropy macrostate of infinite 'energy' that we call our infinite universe. Proto-energy is not Julian Huxley's 1926 *élan locomotif* (locomotive force), which he used to troll the quackery of eighteenth-to-twentieth century *vitalism* as the explication for the force animating Living beings until mechanistic reductionism identified reasons seemingly more plausible for life. Rather, proto-energy is the 'energy' of nature even more primal than the fundamental force lauded by science.

3.2.2 'On–off' Proto-energy

Proto-energy presents as an 'on–off' phenomenon. There is no point space—a single mathematical point in space described by three coordinates relative to an origin—with respect to proto-energy because it's without time and space thus without distance, hence, travel (*SOL* § 6.11.4:198). This is the reason that quantum entanglement appears to science to be instantaneous across the lab or the universe. It's also the reason that Intentional healing works on your body 'instantaneously' (defined on page 109) even at a distance rather than over the course of the days, weeks, months, or years of so-called natural healing. . . or no healing at all.

If we think of a point space in the universe, the proto-energy there is either 'on' or 'off' at any given moment of point-space time. 'On' is when proto-energy is exerting. 'Off' is when it's not. This is to say that 'on' *affects* point space and any matter therein whereas 'off' doesn't, where *affect* means that matter in motion, as archí always are, only interacts with proto-energy when it's 'on.' This is similar to Intentional healing only working when your subconscious is exerting Intentional energy; in other words, it's 'on.' Proto-energy's 'on' phenomenon happens trillions of times a second. It 'moves' and 'undulates' when a point-space region is 'on' at the same time. This means that, instead of proto-energy in any given point space of our physical universe randomly 'on' or 'off,' the whole point-space region is 'on.' It thus exerts with respect to—affecting—the point space and its matter. We liken this to the sound of conversation in a crowd periodically but randomly peaking and falling silent.

From a healing perspective, when you're exerting Intentional energy for the purpose of healing your body, that Intentional energy motivates the proto-energy always suffusing your body to be 'on' and therefore affecting—healing—your whole body or the body part on which you're Intentionally focused. This is because healing isn't simply thinking healing or intoning a mantra, but literally *exerting* 'energy' to affect the point space which, in this case, is your whole body or body part. This sort of 'on–off' oscillation is an aspect of the Way of Being of our universe. It's therefore the Way of Being of Intentional healing since our universe arises in the Intentional mind of its builder interacting with the fundamental essence that is Energent–prime proto-energy.

Matter generically and the 'stuff' of matter is matter–Energy (mE; see CH. 2 § 3.3:65). When the Energent interacts with matter–Energy, the proto-energy involved takes on 'mass'—inertia and the matter side of mE—because now it's no longer simply 'energy' but fundamental force, what Mina calls *real energy*. It is otherwise without 'mass.' The various aspects of fundamental force express in their own subatomic, matter–Energy contexts. The 'energy' to build matter comes from fundamental force reactions with the Energent. This is *applied energy*. But it's the Energent's reaction to the presence of matter–Energy that underwrites it all.

Accordingly, when exerted Intentional energy interacts with proto-energy, it takes on 'mass' in the sense of your Intentionalized Thought. This is because it's now no longer simply 'energy' but Intentionalized by Thought, which Mina calls Intentionalized proto-energy. In other words, via Intentionality the proto-energy suffusing your body or body part *is* the 'energy' of your Intentionalized Thought. For the purpose of healing, it's the original—emergent—Way of Being of your body or body part. The matter–Energy that *is* your body or body part reacts to this Intentionalized proto-energy to, itself, become the 'energy' that *is* emergent Way of Being.

It therefore manifests a healed state, what people call healing. It heals because when the 'energy' of your body *is* the 'energy' of emergent Way of Being, then necessarily it reflects emergent Way of Being which people call perfect health. We cover this in greater detail in Chapter 6.

The value of this section's information is that it helps you understand the infinite reality in which you live and therefore the infinite reality of mind and the presence of 'energy' that your mind interacts with to heal your body. In its essence, it's the very 'energy' of our universe: the Energent. It emanates from the fundamental 'energy'—proto-energy—that is Energent–prime, thus, All Existence. In reorienting your thoughts to comprehend existence in this way, you can liberate your mind from beliefs that limit it. You accordingly empower your ability to heal your body via the Intentional power that is an aspect of your *emergent self-aware proto-energy self*. We touched on that concept in CH. 1 YOU AS A SELF-AWARE PROTO-ENERGY BEING on page 2. Let's briefly reconsider it in the context of the Energent.

3.2.3 You as Emergent ℒife

Emergent ℒife, from which mind constitutes, is ℒife proto-energy, an emergent, self-aware aspect of Energent–prime. Thus, Energent–prime is to psyche (consciousness) as All Existence is to mind. Mind is an emergent of psyche in the same way that All Existence is an emergent of Energent–prime. Psyche is its own Energent except it's self-aware, conscious. In practical terms, it's a self-aware Energent that we call ℒife.

Psyche thus has all the 'energy' potential and capability of Energent–prime which underlies our universe as well as All Existence. It's everything proto-energy is, except that it's self-aware whereas proto-energy is not (SOL § 6.11.4:198). The upshot is that you're essentially a self-aware All Existence. Our psyche transcends the merely existing to the purposed formulating of reality where reality isn't what we *think* it is—how we perceive it—but what we *make* it (SOL § 5.2.1:297). This is why your mind can physically affect what exists in our universe.

Humanity simply hasn't yet experienced the full scope of the human mind. Recall that mind is unlimited, indeterminate, infinite. Accordingly, it's impossible to experience every aspect of mind. About 99.996% of mind is what Philosophy with a capital-P loosely calls subconscious. We're virtually unaware of it, yet it constitutes an individual's who-ness, their absolute self. No matter how much more awareness of mind one develops, there yet remains infinite unawareness (SOL § 2.1.1.1:368). See Chapter 3 for a fuller discussion on you as emergent self-aware proto-energy.

3.2.4 Conclusion to Fundamental Energent

If you're feeling lost in the weeds of scientific gobbledygook, try to see this section as pungent flowers through which you can take in the aroma of all that our universe, and consequently your life, has to offer.

For example, we often aren't aware of all the chemistry and biology behind plant growth. But we plant a flower with the expectation it will grow. Similarly, we haven't known how human life comes to be nor how the world works. Yet, we nonetheless have children and function in the world regardless our lack of comprehension. Allow the fullness of ℒife to unfold for you like flowering petals or a growing child.

3.3 Physical Universe Energies

A brief aside on matter–Energy is in order, as it's an unfamiliar concept and plays an important role in understanding our human environment in which Intentional healing of the body occurs. Note that while mass, mass–energy, and matter–Energy are different, they all reference a tangible, physical object that Philosophy with a capital-P calls matter. First, let's define energy.

3.3.1 Energy

There are three energy types overall: 1) real, actual 'energy' that exerts a presence in reality independent of anything else; 2) 'energy' that exerts in relationships; and 3) measured, or applied, energy that results from those relationships. The first is proto-energy, which is Energent–prime as well as the Energent of our universe. The second is fundamental force. The third is potential, kinetic, inertial, centrifugal, gravitational (weight), and so on. The second expresses in terms of force, such as forces of nature. For science, this includes electromagnetic force, strong/weak nuclear force, and gravity, which doesn't actually exist because it's only a measurement of force in relationship—think of this energy like the energy in a judo throw. An example is $E=mc^2$. Matter (m) and force (F) are applied energy, and are twin *expressions* of the Energent.

As Carnegie-Mellon puts it, "Matter and force are the two fundamental entities of which the universe is composed. All that exists can be classified in these terms. All environmental phenomena occur because of the interactions between matter and transformations of matter in space and time. As the arrangements between forces and masses change, the change is manifested in terms of energy" (SOL § 2.1:114).

Even so, standard as well as quantum science doesn't account for actual 'energy,' such as that which powers fundamental force and life. The Energent is *creation 'energy'* that powers, or enlivens, all (nonhuman) things. Fundamental force is *real energy* that builds matter. We denote it with the Greek uppercase letter Υ (pronounced, *upsilon*). Force generically is *applied energy*, which we denote with the usual symbol E (*see* SOL § 2:114 for a full discussion).

3.3.2 Matter (of Which Your Body Is Made)

Simply stated, matter is the stuff that composes our physical reality, from the tiniest subatomic entity to the largest accretion and includes your physical body. Matter is not simply accumulated stuff like nonliving rock or living tissue because all of that constitutes of archí (literally, encapsulated 'energy;' *below*), which is altogether 'energy,' real energy Υ, and energy in relationship (applied energy E, *above*). Therefore, matter is properly understood as energy, not simply as clumps of stuff. This is why we use the term *matter–Energy* to reference matter.

With respect to the matter–¢nergy (CH. 2 § 3.3.3.1:68) relationship that's familiar to science, an important distinction holds between force and 'energy.' The latter references a certain aspect of the Energent's proto-energy whereas force references proto-energy's interaction with matter that expresses as fundamental force. This came into existence as an expression of the Energent; as soon as the Energent existed then naturally so, too, did fundamental force. In a practical sense, fundamental force is the Energent reactively manifesting to matter, or more accurately, to the 'energy' intrinsic of matter; hence, the term matter–Energy. As a force, then, fundamental force is essentially an Energent force. Prior to matter's existence, fundamental force was simply unexpressed by the Energent's 'energy' flux; a potential force if you will.

When you physically heal your body, you're Intentionally applying 'energy' to the matter—atoms, molecules, cells, tissues—of your body to transform the 'energy' intrinsic to it. This works because matter isn't simply stuff. It's matter–Energy.

3.3.2.1 Archí

As used in *The Story of Life*, archí is a Greek word pronounced *ar-kee* meaning principle, beginning, outset, inception, origin, basis. Think of archí as the *material* version of the *immaterial* Energent. Following the initial inception of our universe, Energent proto-energy emergently coalesced into stable, super 'dense,' ultra-'charged,' self-contained emboli—imagine air bubbles in near-boiling water that don't pop—that segregated from the surrounding 'energy' flux. Each emergent embolus reached sufficient real energy Υ 'charge' and 'density' as to be impermeable to the Energent as well as to other emergent emboli. In so doing, it achieved a construal, tangible physical form—though, at the subatomic, nothing really behaves in the usual corporeal sense—and transitioned in behavior from proto-energy to matter–Energy (matter).

Emergence of matter–Energy doesn't happen with respect to Energent–prime, the proto-energy of All Existence. Rather, it's a unique aspect of the Energent of our universe arising in its Intentional instantiation as an aspect of All Existence. Even though the Energent of our universe *is* Energent–prime, in the context of our universe it exhibits an Intentionalized Way of Being that Energent–prime does not, the purpose of which is to bring into existence a tangible, or *embodied*, universe 'out of' intangible, or *unembodied*, All Existence. This explains our nomenclature making this distinction between the Energent as the proto-energy intrinsic of our universe having *Intentionalized* Way of Being and Energent–prime as the proto-energy of All Existence necessarily having only *emergent* Way of Being.

Archí is the original, irreducible subatomic particle. It's what science terms a truly neutral particle. It weakly emerges continually from the Energent reminiscent of hematopoiesis (formation of blood cells) in bone marrow, concomitantly serving as a metaphorical stem cell for complex matter. An archí necessarily pairwise bonds with another, sufficiently close, archí to form a stable existent that bonds with other bonded archí to form aggregate matter, from the smallest subatomic particle to stars. If an archí fails to pairwise bond within a certain timeframe, it dephases back to proto-energy in the 'energy' flux of the Energent (*SOL* § 2.3.1:115; *see also* the analogy between archí and ℒife in CH. 2 § 2.1.1:35).

3.3.3 Existent 'Energy'

In our universe, the Energent is the root of it all. The Energent is life—not ℒife itself, of course, but the presence behind (nonhuman) life that gives physical things motility and the ability to be. My daughters and I wanted to call it *energy* when we learned about it but it's just not (*SOL* § 4.3:150). It mandates a fundamental rethink to cognize its existential nature, but that's a whole nother tale in *The Story of ℒife* (CH. 17:111). As a conceptual baseline, Mina selected the term *enérgeia*, a Greek word for action, act, or work in terms of energy. He uses it in the sense of "the energetic essentiality of a thing's nature," and likens it to Aristotle's view that *enérgeia* is not a movement (*kinēsis*), since it has no endpoint of completion. Rather, that what's happening is happening in a complete way in and of itself (else it's not happening at all): "Every moment of... consciousness is a perfect whole" (Rackham (c. 353–322 BC) 1956, x.4.1174b, 593–5).

Enérgeia is not applied energy E nor real energy Υ nor the Energent. Applied energy E describes energy as motion, force, or work that results *from* real energy Υ, nature's empowering force. The Energent, *enérgeia*'s parent, is the "absolute essentiality of a thing's nature" in our universe like *its* parent Energent-prime in All Existence. Let's more closely define *enérgeia*.

3.3.3.1 *Enérgeia*

Enérgeia manifests from the interaction between matter and Energent. Ultimately, *a thing—a piece of matter*—isn't Energent but *material* Energent. Here lies true matter–¢nergy (*below*) equivalence: a thing embodies *enérgeia*, manifests real energy Υ, and operates as applied energy E. The full spectrum of existence *in* our universe rises from the Energent to (natural *or* supranatural) matter like the alpha and omega *of* our universe.

We capitalize Energy in matter–Energy to distinguish it from the conventional matter–energy that science uses (which we typeset as matter–¢nergy for clarity) because what science calls energy is actually applied energy. Einstein's matter–¢nergy equivalence, expressed as $E=mc^2$, is really a mass–applied energy relationship. Mass, however, is an insufficient concept to understand energy equivalence. $E=mc^2$ isn't equivalent to 'energy' generally but to applied energy specifically. His formula simply means that *energy is equivalent to mass in motion*. Hence, $E=mc^2$ is really saying that motion energy is *equivalent* to matter in motion ($\overleftrightarrow{E} = \overleftrightarrow{m}$). Consequently, mass as a convention to comprehend real energy equivalence needs replacing by matter–Energy for the reasons we discuss in SOL § 2:114.

Enérgeia is the Energent's *expression* in time and space; the Energent itself has no time and space (CH. 2 § 3.2.2:62; SOL § 6.11.4:198; it is the proto-energy 'inside' the archí constituting its entirety). Overall, the Energent omnidirectionally '*moves*' and '*undulates*' like a lake with many agitation vectors whereas *enérgeia* multidirectionally '*flows*' such as through inter-archí spaces (SOL § 6.9.3.3:182). Energent proto-energy and *enérgeia* are different. *Enérgeia* is 'energy' that forms on the fly 'out of' proto-energy in response to the motion of matter (matter–Energy) 'through' the Energent. It is proto-energy's flux across matter giving rise to *enérgeia* that creates real energy Υ (fundamental force) from which arises applied energy E. Nowhere in the infinite universe is matter—even a single, pairwise archí—too insufficient for *enérgeia* to manifest (*SOL* § 4.3:150).

When you or another are healing your physical body, the proto-energy that *is* Intentional Thought Intentionalizes the proto-energy suffusing your body or body part. The *enérgeia* arising in this context as described above is thus the 'energy' of emergent Way of Being, which is what you're Intentionalizing: perfect health. *Enérgeia* is what transforms your body or body part from the 'energy' of damage—illness, disease, injury, aging—to the 'energy' of emergent Way of Being. The matter–Energy of your body or body part responds to this *enérgeia*. As it more and more fully responds to it, your body or body part *is* this 'energy' instead of the 'energy' of damage and, therefore, *is* perfect health.

3.4 Conclusion to the Milieu in Which Your Body Lives

Our universe exists as a discrete, infinite entity in the context of All Existence, which is 'all there infinitely is.' Although our universe is infinite it doesn't, by definition, include All Existence. Energent–prime proto-energy is the 'energy' of All Existence whereas Energent proto-energy, which is the same 'energy' despite Mina Intentionalizing it in the creation process of our universe, *is* the 'energy' that powers all things of our universe. It's the difference between the former as an emergent property and the latter as Intentionality. This 'energy' includes your physical body but not you the emergently birthed, self-aware proto-energy person who exists separate and apart from our universe albeit not All Existence. The Energent is the root of fundamental force and applied energy E in our universe; science generally comprehends this as energy. Chapter 17 in *The Story of Life* is a comprehensive dissertation on All Existence and 'energy' that you might want to give a shot. For now, we turn our attention to our mind and body.

Section 4
Mind and Body

Recall that Living is the state of aliveness in nonhuman life whereas human life is Life and there is no other Life than Human. Also, that the physically alive person is first and foremost mind, which is entirely nonphysical in every sense of the word; it integrates the physical body so as to interact with and experience the physical environment of our universe. To understand mind in the context of its physical embodiment, we need first briefly describe 𝕃iving brain. The reason is that the human brain, unlike 𝕃iving brain, operates on two fundamental levels. First, it's a 𝕃iving entity. Second, it's an integrator of the body with the ℘erson . . . not the instantiated mind of 𝕃iving brain, but the *self* as emergent ℒife.

4.1 Nonhuman Mind–Brain–Body

We describe the human mind–brain–body in CH. 2 § 4.2:72. Here, we describe 𝕃iving nonhuman (animal) mind as it operates through the brain–body matrix. Although the human body (not the person) is a 𝕃iving entity that's fundamentally no different from albeit certainly more brain sophisticated than any other animal except the elephant, the human brain, unlike other 𝕃iving entity brains, integrates autonomous ℒife mind. It's a unique case and described in detail in *The Story of ℒife* § 1.2.2:253ff. Even so, from a sans-ℒife-mind-brain-only perspective, this section applies to the human brain as well.

Philosophy with a capital-P's reductionist effort—from neuroscience to psychology and all points between—to understand the mind–body problem and generate a useful conceptual comprehension of mind has ended up largely describing 𝕃iving (animal) mind while entirely missing the boat on ℒife (human) mind. The reason is simple: its focus on function over instantiation. Since each instantiated human mind is unique with respect to any other instantiation, mind isn't reducible to function, especially brain function. About 75% of 𝕃iving entities have a distributed intelligence mind with the remainder possessing a brain mind (SOL Table 5:235). It's to the latter we now turn.

4.1.1 Instantiation of Nonhuman Mind

𝕃iving—nonhuman—mind is an emergent property of brain (SOL § 2:90). That doesn't mean it's a "self-organizing property of energy and information flow as it unfolds" (Siegel 2016, 2:8) in and about the brain–body. Nor that it's "an information processing system . . . translating changes in the body and the environment into a language of neural impulses that represent the animal-environment relationship . . . [as] information instantiated in and processed by the nervous system" (Henriques 2011, par. 5). These are *functional* definitions. Mind is rather a moment-by-moment *emergent* macro instantiation of hundreds of trillions of *non-emergent* yet self-organizing micro *instantiations of awareness* that begin as somatic or nonsomatic experiences of environment.

A somatic experience is a neuroresponse to a state of being in or around the body's environment (SOB is one's experience of the referent state of awareness (SOA), i.e., the awareness that one has in totality with respect to what's of interest; *see* CH. 4:119). A nonsomatic experience is a neuroresponse to an instantiation of awareness (SOA) at less than the macro level. Indeed, a nonsomatic experience at the macro level qualifies as a rudimentary, self-existing-mind self-awareness. Living entities entirely lack this although higher-order animals do exhibit a faux self-awareness. This means they have no awareness of self-awareness, instead having self-unawareness. The latter is the ability to subjectively reflect on objective reality *without* awareness that they are subjectively experiencing objective reality (*see* SOL § 2.2:278 for greater detail). In other words, they are not self-aware that they *are* self-aware, whereas humans have awareness *of* self-awareness.

An informational (or, data flow) emergent property resides in being a novel interaction amongst data. It therefore exists as an emergent existent where the many micro states of awareness from which it instantiates are the product of novel, supervenient—unexpected—interactions of predictable outcomes of brain activity or information flow. This emergent existent makes Living mind a weakly emergent property of proto-energy's interaction with the electromagnetic (EM) nature of each *action potential*—the electrochemical nerve impulse originating in the brain and body instantiated from Energent proto-energy's interaction with the matter–Energy of neuronal and somatic activity—and its micro-SOA and their coalescence into expanding collections of states of awareness. This altogether results in the emergent generation of a real Energent proto-energy existent, i.e., animal mind. It's an 'energy' field, though not one of applied energy E such as electromagnetic, thermal, and so on.

Each micro-SOA—every neuronal impulse—alters the whole such that Living mind instantiates and reinstantiates moment-to-moment as a discrete proto-energy existent—animal mind—so long as the brain experiences action potentials (SOL § 1.2.2:253). This means Living mind is a discrete reality *emergently transcending* brain even while it draws its moment-to-moment existence from it. Thus, when Living brain dies then so, too, dissipates Living mind. This outcome more or less aligns with Philosophy with a capital-P's theories of materialism and physicalism except that, in conflating Living (animal) mind—in the context of having consciousness—with Life (human) mind, these theories are wholly inaccurate therefore inadequate.

4.1.2 Nonhuman Brain–body Integration

The nonhuman 𝕃iving entity having some level of brain—animal, insect—operates its body through a neural interface. This means action potentials not only *in the brain* but *throughout the body* like a wiring harness. Nerve impulses inform the brain of sensory input, which processes it and sends neural impulses back. An example would be an animal touching a burning surface. The brain responds to sensory neural input with motor signals that cause the animal to jerk away from the source of damage.

No matter how sophisticated the nonhuman brain—this applies to the proto-human brain prior to 𝔥uman integration during the evolutionary period from its primitive origin (SOL § 2:542)—it is a *neural entity*, not a *being of mind*. It's entire awareness of and experience with life happens by and through its neural interface with its environment regardless sophistication. This is not the case with the 𝔥uman-integrated body. We consider this aspect in CH. 2 § 4.3.2:77.

4.2 Human Mind–Brain–Body

We reiterate that, unlike 𝕃iving brain, the human brain operates on two fundamental levels. First, as a 𝕃iving entity. Second, as an integrator of the body with the person; not the instantiated mind of 𝕃iving brain (SOL § 1.3.2:273) but the self as emergent ℒife.

As a 𝕃iving entity, our brain *at the present time* functions essentially the same as any nonhuman 𝕃iving entity in terms of somatic sensation, nerve impulses, and instantiated mind. It differs, however, in that its instantiated—meaning, emergent—mind operates in a ℒife environment of real, which is to say self-existing, mind... as a 𝔭erson. Whereas a 𝕃iving entity's instantiated mind is the apex of its subjective sensory integration with its objective environment, mind instantiated by the human brain operates autonomously in tandem with a person's ℒife mind. Let's look at this instantiated physical mind before describing how it integrates ℒife mind.

4.2.1 Physical Mind as Facsimile of ℒife Mind

Your brain is just an electrochemical processor. Its magic happens when Energent proto-energy interacts with its matter–Energy constituents to instantiate physical mind as a weak emergent albeit not as a *working*, i.e., nonhuman, mind since it doesn't think, feel, or act *itself*. Put differently,

② Physical Mind as Facsimile of 𝓛ife Mind

animal (𝕃iving) mind *is* animal brain. Human mind is *not* human brain, it is 𝓛ife mind integrating brain. Recall that *weak* emergence is an emergent property (e.g., formation of a traffic jam; structure of a flock in flight or a school of fish; formation of galaxies) that's theoretically reducible to causal accounts of its elementary parts retaining their independence whereas *strong* emergence is an emergent property that's not even theoretically reducible to its elementary parts; it is *novel*.

The truly fascinating thing about humans' physical mind is that it's a physically emergent facsimile of 𝓛ife mind; in other words, *you*. 𝓛ife mind is what folks often imagine as their spirit mind or spirit self, their *true* self. 𝓛ife mind is emergent proto-energy. It's therefore unable to interact directly on its unembodied own with either the natural or supranatural environments of a universe. Physical mind, on the other hand, is an Energent proto-energy emergent expression of a person's 𝓛ife mind. Since 𝓛ife mind integrates brain, it naturally integrates brain's panoply of micro and macro states of being and states of awareness, in effect *integrating* instantiated physical mind which is the macro state of awareness and state of being of brain. Recall, too, that state(s) of awareness (SOA) refers to the awareness one has in totality with respect to what's of interest, and state(s) of being (SOB) is one's experience of the referent SOA.

Instantiated physical mind is a collective term for holistic Energent proto-energy that makes up the vast micro and macro state(s) of being and state(s) of awareness that comprise your brain's overall macro-SOA, which reflects both 𝓛ife mind's nonphysical state(s) of awareness and brain's physical state(s) of awareness. That's what instantiated physical mind really is: *a dynamic, emergent, macro-SOA instantiation of proto-energy in the context of the physical environment* . . . an invisible 'energy' existent.

𝓛ife mind isn't just magically 'aware' of every state of being and state of awareness incident to your body. 'Energy' is the vehicle through which awareness happens. Your body's every physicochemical experience translates via matter–Energy to Energent proto-energy. At each step, this proto-energy expresses the micro-SOB and a micro-SOA built up from your physical self's every archí constituent interacting with proto-energy which generates fundamental force that, in turn, generates electromagnetism and other applied energy E forces. These applied energy E instantiations themselves interact with proto-energy to constitute the referenced micro and macro state(s) of being and state(s) of awareness.

If one could visually observe the proto-energy suffused in and around a person's physical body, one would see a kaleidoscope of ever-changing

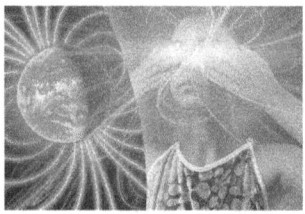

Fig. 2.3. Consider your physically instantiated mind as analogous to Earth's electromagnetic (geomagnetic) field. The difference is that the 'energy' of your physically instantiated mind remains within the brain instead of forming a field beyond the brain as with Earth's geomagnetic field.[2]

'energy' fields, patterns, strengths, extensions, and so on. Any physical entity is a constantly shifting expression of proto-energy, real energy Υ (fundamental force), and applied energy E (kinetic, motion, electromagnetic, and binding 'energies'). This is what thinkers are getting at when they say the human body is energy; that *you* are energy. But it's inadequate, as it lacks awareness of 'energy.'

So, how is our ℒife proto-energy mind—our real, emergently eternal self—aware of all this? Well, it 'reads'—encounters—all these 'energies' expressed as Energent proto-energy and comprehends—experiences—it all in the state-of-being and state-of-awareness terms it understands via the physical body's integration with the spirit body which itself manifests ℒife mind in the 'reflective' environment. Recall that the 'reflective' is a sort of natural–supranatural 'border' area wherein the physical person interacts with the spirit environment. This is how our ℒife mind is just 'aware' of what's going on with our physical self in our physical environment from which, by its nature, it's somatically excluded. It isn't any different, really, than a radio receiver plucking invisible energy out of the ether through the principles described by physics, yet expressing—comprehending—it in audio, or in television's audiovisual, terms.

For example, a nominal action potential (AP) is more than just a ±40 millivolt (mv) electrical charge with an attendant electromagnetic (EM) field of charge, polarity, strength, frequency, and so on. Each action potential represents an electromagnetic field that's unique in toto albeit having certain constituents that integrate—are the same as—those of certain other action potentials. This means that such action potentials are EM field-relevant to each other and thereby form a *clade*.

A clade is a taxonomic designation for biological *taxa*—a group of organisms that form a unit—that share features inherited from a common ancestor. Here, we use clade in the context of brain. Take, for instance, the many individual somatic neuroresponses (e.g., temperature, pain) occasioned by touching a hot surface. They share certain EM field elements common to the experience which the brain then processes, categorizes, experiences, and so on as a clade it then relates to own-self wellbeing.

This means individual neuroresponses that are EM-field related dynamically group via neural processes as they move through your brain's neural pathways. Accordingly, an action potential is really just a vehicle for moving an EM field to where it can integrate other relevant EM fields . . . not too unlike what molecular motor proteins (*actin*) do in their own context to convert chemical energy to mechanical work in order to 'walk' along actin filaments to contract muscles or along intracellular microtubules to move 'cargo' (Yildiz 2024). This altogether instantiates, in applied energy E terms, the Energent proto-energy that expresses a particular micro-SOA and macro-SOA of our brain in conjunction with our ℒife mind.

The brain experiences and comprehends nothing more than electrochemical action potentials, each of which expresses a unique 'data point.' Because we are self-aware ℒife, we find it difficult if not impossible to comprehend how a brain—a 𝕃iving entity—experiences the world. Does a brain think, and if so, how? While it's an amazingly capable instrument, the brain doesn't experience Thought (thinking–feeling), which is the exclusive province of ℒife mind. The human brain *mimics* Thought because it transliterates ℒife mind into a physically instantiated, or facsimile, mind. *Transliterate* means to convert ℒife mind's direct awareness into cognition, or brainspeak, similar in some respects to the way that software transliterates computer binary code into human-comprehensible language. The nonhuman (non-ℒife-mind-integrated) brain doesn't think although it does (non-emotively) feel because action potentials can only convey neuroresponse. Thus, on its own, brain merely instantiates an experience that's redolent—in the sense of expressive—with impression because feeling, in this context, is fundamentally impression not emotion.

This is true of course for humans, too, as our brain is a 𝕃iving, nonhuman entity. This goes unnoticed because, as emergent ℒife, we can think-feel and our brain integrates ℒife mind's Thought with our physical self. Even so, we're fundamentally (emotively) feeling beings. The way that we experience own-self state of being is emotive (consciously or subconsciously), meaning in a way that's redolent with impression. Consciously thinking is our unique ability to parse feeling's impression into a particular state of awareness that we physically cognize and can analyze in the context of human self-awareness. The nature of feeling comprises most of our thought, with only about 0.01% comprising thinking (*SOL* § 4.2:292). This is the difference between our subconscious and conscious minds.

4.3 Mind–body Integration

Just as our spirit and physical bodies integrate, so, too, does our (emergent ℒife) spirit and physical (brain-instantiated) mind. Our spirit, or ℒife, mind doesn't emanate from any sort of spirit brain, as no such anatomy exists in our spirit body unless we choose to manifest it. Even so, spirit-born persons feel their seat of consciousness—their mind, their *personness*—in their head much as physical-born persons do (there are obvious dissimilarities, but we don't discuss them in this book nor in *The Story of ℒife*). It's part of ℒife's intrinsic Way of Being. Since ℒife mind manifests the spirit body, then anywhere that body is, so is one's mind. Consequently, spirit–physical body integration, which we call physicospirit, means spirit–physical mind integration. As physical (instantiated) mind is an Energent proto-energy existent of brain, the real integration going on here is between spirit (ℒife) mind and physical brain.

With integration, spirit mind *is* physical brain and physical brain *is* spirit mind. They are (ideally) one and the same. Even though discrete and autonomous, and notwithstanding the dichotomy described above, there's no substantive difference between them as an integration. One is the other notwithstanding mind–brain integration disruptions occasioned by The Corruption. But they do operate differently.

The brain is built around cognitively processing micro-SOA via nerve impulses plus mind as direct awareness. To that end, transliteration needs happen to convert mind's direct awareness into brainspeak as noted in CH. 2 § 4.2.1 on page 72. Neurons do this work. In the nonhuman brain, neurons experience action potentials strictly as somatic phenomena. Humans operate in an entirely different environment, one that includes the physical but transcends it as well. This is why the most sophisticated nonhuman can never glimpse even the most mundane human experience howsoever they mimic it or humans attempt to train them. The difference is literally rocks to food. However, mind–body integration differs significantly from mind–brain integration, so let's consider it.

4.3.1 Self-awareness

Self-awareness comes from how mind encounters stimuli. It doesn't process stimuli, because mind isn't cognitive but assimilative (SOL § 1:391). This means we don't simply encounter stimuli and then cognize it in order to objectively or subjectively experience it. Mind is unstructured and energetic, not structured and procedural. Conversely, the brain has procedural structure to process data input and output in order to integrate cognitive body to assimilative mind. Essentially, it's a transliteration processor.

What science presumes to be human brain cognition is simply the brain engaged in transliteration processing as well as own-self brain–body sensory and regulatory functions. In this respect, it's essentially an 'avatar.' Brain works very much like a computer's random access memory (RAM) with limited storage capacity. So long as the brain is alive, whatever it stores remains until 'overwritten' by *brainstate reinstantiation*, the constant updating of physically instantiated mind some 1,000 times per second via integrated ℒife mind (*SOL* § 1.2.2.4.2.1:258).

All else being normal, brain capacity rises and falls according to the demands that mind places on it. This resolves the mystery of how the brain, which is plainly structurally limited, appears limitless in capacity and capability (*SOL* § 2.1:276): all of our thinking–feeling originates as a wholistic state of being and state of awareness in the subconscious that Intentionalizes literally infinite such states to the conscious mind where we parse them into 𝕋hought. Subconscious awareness is not only too fast for our brain to operate on, but its mode of awareness is incompatible with brain's functionality of cognition. Transliteration is thus required from one environment to the other (*SOL* § 2.1:393).

Because we aren't our bodies, one can never compare human to non-human based on shared physicality. That's like comparing the *driver* of a car to other *cars*. This lack of awareness of what really comprises human is what trips up Philosophy with a capital-P to draw immaterial conclusions about human beings based on evolutionary, genetic, and related analyses of the 𝕃iving physical body that frustratingly clash with our deeper sensibilities and lived experience that involve our ℒife self.

The Corruption interfered with mindset and, ultimately, mind–brain and mind–body integration, meaning transliteration. We experience a mental blindness as well as a structural limitation in the brain that limits our physically instantiated mind's self-awareness and how much of it can integrate the brain at any given moment (*SOL* § 1.2.2.5:261). The practical result is that we're cut off from the fullness of ℒife and unable to experience most of our own states of awareness. This isn't a permanent condition, however (*SOL* § 2.1:393; *SOL* CH. 24:361).

4.3.2 Human Mind–body Integration

Science currently sees the human brain operating its body through a neural interface like a wiring harness just as we saw with nonhuman brain–body integration. Nerve impulses inform the brain of sensory input which processes it and sends neural impulses back. We use the previous example but with a human touching a burning surface. The brain responds to sensory neural input with motor signals that cause the body to jerk away from the source of damage. This forms today's prevailing understanding of the human body's essential function and operation. Lacking any awareness of human physicospirit reality, Philosophy with a capital-P presumes the human body *thus the person* is naught but a smarter, cleverer, übersophisticated animal. This is entirely inaccurate, however, as the person—being a ℘erson—is a *being of mind*, not a *neural entity*.

The reason our bodies appear to function and operate as merely animal lies in The Corruption severing our awareness of human physicospirit reality from the get-go about 50,000 years ago (SOL § 2:542). This left us adrift in a material environment that, despite our very imperfect, residual awareness of spirit existence, emphasized only one reality: matter. It is true that our *essential* (as opposed to *full*) awareness of and experience with life primarily happens by and through our neural interface with our environment regardless how sophisticated our spirit awareness. But that's our physically instantiated self's Way of Being *today*, not our physicospirit self's Way of Being *originally*.

Recall that mind–*body* integration is *of* the subconscious whereas mind–*brain* integration is subconscious–conscious. Subconscious (an aspect of your proto-energy self) integrates your body wholistically such that the body *is* your subconscious. There is no distinction. This is why our bodies get sick, age, and die despite our conscious aversion to all three. They are the *attributive habits* of our subconscious thus our body's attributive Way of Being. Our subconscious accepts as real that the body is animal, a neural entity. In its unawareness of the 'energy' of emergent Way of Being, our body consequently manifests via subconscious Intentionality all the accoutrements of a 𝕃iving entity. This dual, neural–mind function and operation is the case even today. But it's not how we originally are.

In our intended physicospirit embodiment *in The Corruption's environment* mind integrates brain, our proto-energy self via subconscious integrates body, and the 'energy' of emergent Way of Being manifests in the matter–Energy of the body throughout. The brain functions and operates via action potentials (neural impulses) as set out in CH. 2 § 4.1.1 on page 70. The body, exclusive of brain, functions and operates via subconscious *amalgamation*, an aspect of integration (in the sense of alloy as an admixture where entities retain their individual properties; CH. 4:119). Your body *is* your proto-energy self (via subconscious) because it, thus your body, is instantly aware of conscious mind. For example, you want to consciously or subconsciously move your arm. Either way, moving it is a subconscious Intentionality. It therefore *is* your physical arm. Your arm accordingly integrates this subconscious Intentionality via brain and moves.

In a sense, subconscious amalgamation of your body *is* the wiring harness that's presently manifested as the neural network that is the body's nervous system. But although your body is a 𝕃iving entity because it is matter–Energy having its own independent Way of Being in the context of the natural environment, the physiological reality that is a 𝕃iving entity's mode of existence is unnecessary to that entity which integrates ℒife—the human person—as a literal extension of mind. As noted, however, the body's nervous system functioning and operating as an extension of brain is merely a manifested result of our unawareness of our physicospirit reality. It exists only because our attributive subconscious Way of Being manifested it in lieu of emergent subconscious Way of Being. With full mind–body integration, a nervous system (including brain) is redundant and irrelevant. In truth, physicospirit awareness means the internal functions of the human body differs so drastically from how it is today as to be unrecognizable. We don't discuss that aspect in this book since healing your body *today* needs be in accord with your body as it *is*.

With this conceptual understanding of your physicospirit reality, you can see why and how it's possible to Intentionally heal your body to perfect health and wellbeing. You simply need let go your attributive subconscious Way of Being so that the 'energy' of emergent Way of Being manifests as the 'energy' of the matter–Energy of your body without interference. Although a healer can transform, or heal, this or that health issue, so long as your subconscious Intentionalizes attributive habits into your body, that transformation will always be temporary. We'll get into this in greater detail beginning with Chapter 3.

Section 5
Infinity of Psyche

Consciousness—logically albeit not materially equivalent to psyche, the totality that is mind where mind is ℘erson—is what we talk about when referencing what's unique, special, or differentiating about being human. On its own, however, 'consciousness' just doesn't capture it. The key thing is that the essence of so-called consciousness is *personness* which is ℌuman, humanness, emergent awareness, and altogether 𝓛ife. Its functions (e.g., freedom, existence, choice, self-awareness, awareness, qualia) are properties of the 𝓹erson. Nonhumans possess the same essence and functionality of entity as humans but aren't 𝔍uman, thus, not having 𝓛ife. This means that nonhuman *aliveness* is 𝕃iving and nonhuman *life* isn't 𝓛ife. Accordingly, nonhumanness—biology—is 𝕃iving not 𝓛ife (*see* SOL CH. 19:245 for a full discussion).

You are infinite mind, not finite brain.

Infinite spirituality, not finite materiality.

An infinite All Existence, not a finite locality of mind.

But what does infinite even mean in the human context? Philosophy with a capital-P has so far only ever described *human* in functional terms. But you aren't a function, are you? You're a being. A self-aware proto-energy person. Accordingly, your true essence is 'energy' not function, and certainly not body. Practically speaking, as a being of 'energy' you are, in your fundamentals, a self-aware All Existence. Where All Existence is infinite, *unaware* proto-energy (in the context of existence), the human person—you—is infinite, *self-aware* proto-energy (in the context of All Existence). Accordingly, we can only describe human *as* Way of Being just as with All Existence.

Yet, we can't describe Way of Being (except its expressions such as self-aware proto-energy where 𝓛ife, 𝔍uman, 𝓹erson, and mind are manifestations of it) because it's proto-energy; it's without time and space. In your humanness you, too, are without time and space. You only think you're a being of time and space, as you emergently birthed integrating a physical body in an environment of time and space. Because of The Corruption, we have nothing more than a vague connection to what we truly are.

Human consciousness—psyche—integrates the one and only Reality that is All Existence, which is 'all there infinitely is' (SOL Eq. 15.13:102). This means that although All Existence is existentially real (integrated but defined by its own Way of Being in which Energent–prime is its distinct aspect, separate and apart from humanity and universes generally), it is merely existence. Its *reality* comes from human consciousness. For example, there is no time infinity with respect to All Existence outside consciousness because time(-keeping), a product of *event periodicity* (*below*), is *of* consciousness (SOL CH. 16:105). Outside of consciousness, there's no time at all. It's nonexistent.

The same goes for space and existence. Each one is infinite—indeterminate—because what consciousness is, itself, *is what they are*. This is why you are what you think and, accordingly, why you can physically heal. A malfunction in your body—illness, disease, damage—is existence, an existentiality. Your experience of it is reality, a subjectivism. Intentionally healing your body changes reality and, therefore, your body's existentiality. Existence is not reality; reality *is* existence.

5.1 Event Periodicity

Besides the momentariness of unbonded archí, event periodicity arises in the elemental motion of the singular albeit bonded archí, the foundational unit of matter–Energy. At its most objectively fundamental, event periodicity is time and time is event periodicity, where event periodicity is materially equivalent to time and thus time is implied by, or presumes, event periodicity. Timekeeping occurs when we settle on some predictable rhythm to regulate our perception—the reality—of event periodicity. A few examples of a predictable rhythm are the resonance of cesium-133 atoms, the oscillations of a quartz crystal, thoughts, feelings, or experiences in blockchain, biological or natural cycles, and so forth.

Outside the human desire to be aware of and establish a regulatory matrix for event periodicity, time is not an existential thing with existent properties. Thus, where the set of all properties of time doesn't exist, there are no such properties, hence, no time. There is only event periodicity at whatever macroscopic or microscopic level whereat events occur (see *sol* § 2:107 for a full discussion).

5.2 Consciousness and Reality

Until now, our universe was the only driver for our sense of the existence of all things. As we earlier noted, however, the Energent, being 'all there infinitely is' *in the context of our universe*, grounds matter and fundamental force. Thus, it's impossible to cognize these two existent aspects of a universe outside that context. And because the Energent itself grounds in Energent–prime, neither can we cognize our universe absent All Existence. Accordingly, and in any case, it isn't possible to consider the existence of our universe properly without grounding it in All Existence.

Neither can we cognize emergent *L*ife sans All Existence (*Fig. 2.4*:83) because *L*ife emergently births 'in' Energent proto-life, which itself is an emergent property of Energent–prime that grounds All Existence. In the same way that trying to comprehend our universe outside the context of All Existence is like investigating what a lightbulb does without considering electricity, we can't understand emergent ℒife absent All Existence for the simple reason that ℒife—*you*—is, effectively, an *emergently self-aware Energent–prime, i.e., an individual All Existence* (*see* page 2). As existents, all these aspects thread the same needle. Everything that exists suffuses 'in' All Existence. There's no understanding anything without understanding that. Existence as existentiality grounds in the singular root of Energent–prime, which grounds All Existence. But Energent–prime (together with All Existence *as* undescribable Way of Being) literally *does not exist* outside consciousness because, of all things that do exist, only consciousness—psyche—has self-awareness that *is* Way of Being.

Therefore, since you are an emergently self-aware All Existence (of proto-energy) in your own right, a malfunction in your body literally *does not exist* outside of your consciousness. Why? Because that malfunction grounds in your Intentional ℒife mind, which 'energy' response to the world Intentionalizes the existence of that malfunction. You experience that malfunction *as* reality. Your subconscious recreates your body's Way of Being to include that malfunction. And the cycle continues. Accordingly, when you remove that malfunction as a reality of your mind you cease Intentionalizing the malfunction as an existence and thereby restore—transform—your body's Way of Being as an existence closer to emergent Way of Being, meaning perfect health. And then you experience *that* reality.

Let's revisit and extend the above lightbulb analogy. Recall that ℒife force is the emergent proto-energy incorporating emergent Way of Being of your self-aware proto-energy self, the *you* that is you. As an analogy, it enlivens—powers—your body similar to electricity enlivening—powering—a lightbulb. Being aware of electricity, people accept that it will always be there to light the bulb, or capable of being there as an infinite force in the universe. Similarly, you don't have to *grow into* ℒife force. You simply need be *aware* of it. Awareness empowers it. Although ℒife force powers your body, physical humanity believes in the reality that only physical forces such as chemistry and biology power it. But that's a presumed reality of existence rooted in our lack of awareness of our emergent birth and physicospirit embodiment.

Moreover, Mina tells us that ℒife force, the very 'energy' that is the human person as a proto-energy being, can theoretically power the universe just as Energent–prime and the Energent do, except that megaversal humanity (including Mike and Molly) never learned how. The reason is that building an Energent–prime-powered universe was discovered first and is apparently easier, besides. For a person to heal a physical body, he or

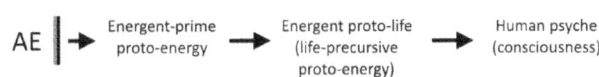

Fig. 2.4. Each iteration of All Existence (AE) emergently arose, not evolved, from a previous AE. Energent proto-life and consciousness emergently arose and birthed, respectively, from Current AE (Chapter 2 § 1.1–1.1.2:26–27).

she needs accept and understand the infinite omniscience, omnipresence, omnipotence, and omniexistence of ℒife force in them as an emergent property of All Existence (this isn't necessary to be healed by a healer).

The distinction between existence as both existentiality and reality is crucial because, until now, you've probably believed with certitude that the malfunctions of your body are natural, normal, inevitable, the will of God, in some cases meant to be or deserved; essentially, the Way of Being of physical humanity. As you can see, when you comprehend the reality of your existence in terms of All Existence and emergent Way of Being, your new reality substantively changes your physical existence.

You can 'instantly' heal yourself when you have awareness of the omniscience, omnipresence, omnipotence, and omniexistence of ℒife force as the 'energy' of your body. That your body is not *matter*, it is *matter-Energy*, which means your body *is* 'energy.' That this 'energy' *is your* ℒife force, which you can manipulate just as you manipulate your own thoughts in your conscious mind and train—habituate—your subconscious. This reality has always been there. You are only now becoming aware of it. Awareness unlocks the power of your mind just as it did for Mike and Molly as they discovered the reality of their own minds in their curious explorations to interact with the other and, eventually, build a universe, embody, and emergently procreate.

Today, people subconsciously block the reality of ℒife force in their body for the reality that biology and physical forces enlivens and controls their body outside the will of their minds. This happens because your (self-aware) proto-energy self is an Intentional machine—it self-actualizes; what you accept as real, you literally make real. Awareness gives you choice. Change your choice, change your reality.

5.3 Omniscience, Omnipresence, Omnipotence, Omniexistence

Throughout the ages, psyche—what's called *consciousness* by Philosophy with a capital-p—was addressed only in the context of our universe. Despite currently living in our universe physically (and spirit) embodied, we don't actually *exist* here because psyche exists as existentiality in the context of All Existence and Energent proto-life, not a universe. *Psyche is extrauniversal.* That might sound initially silly, but consider that 𝓛ife—you, the individual—is fundamentally an emergently self-aware All Existence. In consequence, 𝓛ife inherits properties such as proto-energy, existence, time, and spatial indeterminance that give rise to attributes hitherto conceptualized only in a deific sense as omniscience, omnipresence, omnipotence, and omniexistence. Here, omniscience means "emergent 𝓛ife awareness of self" that arises from a knowingness of self about which it's necessarily impossible to be mistaken (SOL § 3:331).

This means it's not possible for emergent 𝓛ife to be confined to exist in only one single place *anywhere* as a *reality*—say, in one's body. The reason is that a person, as mind, literally exists in all places *everywhere* as existentiality via awareness. This is the case even though, strange as it seems, one exists *nowhere* as nondimensional—without time and space—existentiality at the same time. Sure, we don't feel very omnipresent all shoeboxed into our physical body. But that's only because our physical embodiment, lacking the balance of being well versed in our spirit embodiment and unembodied fundamentality, has inured our minds to this and only this limited reality. We'll say it again: you are not your body, physical *or* spiritual. *You are mind.*

Although the implication of this notion appears to be that one exists and doesn't exist at the same time like Schrödinger's infamous cat, it's not a contradiction because the combination of existence as existentiality and reality necessarily means that one exists regardless reality and one has reality regardless existence. We don't appreciate this caveat with respect to our universe, which existence *is* Way of Being *with* matter–Energy that gives rise naturally to empirical observation and reasoning. But it's clear with respect to All Existence, which existence *is* Way of Being *without* matter–Energy that, despite existing as existentiality (and unlike a universe), we can't perceive exists except as reality, meaning as an experiential existent... an existence we experience via 𝓛ife mind.

What this means in regards to 𝓛ife is that, while we exist as existentiality, we can't *perceive* we exist except as reality. Unlike Descartes' *cogito, ergo sum* ("I think, therefore I am," which presumes the conclusion, the means, *and* subjective existence), *in perceiving, there is perception* which, in and of itself, is an existent but only one that's percepted; there is existence as reality. To get at existence as existentiality, one needs perceive Way of Being.

This section conceptually exposes emergent 𝓛ife's Way of Being such that we can perceive human existence as existentiality. This is to say that,

OMNISCIENCE, OMNIPRESENCE, OMNIPOTENCE, OMNIEXISTENCE

as a self-aware proto-energy being, a person is everywhere yet, suffused 'in' nondimensional Energent proto-life, is simultaneously nowhere (*SOL* § 2.3.2.1:241). On the other hand, as percepted reality, wherever your mind is, wherever you're aware, there you are. Wherever you're not aware, there you're not.

Your body is merely an integration whereby nondimensional mind integrates dimensional environment such as, for instance, how an interface integrates components with a user or a vehicle integrates a driver with travel. Through your integrated body you, having mind, can phenomenally experience an environment outside of mind. Your *body* exists here (and in spirit world). However, your *mind* exists everywhere yet nowhere as existentiality and, although *present* as reality where your body is, it can be present as reality anywhere because of its existence *as* existentiality. Indeed, one can be present simultaneously in more than one context, meaning in more than one reality (*SOL* § 1.2.3.3.3:472).

We exist nowhere because our place of existence and our existentiality as emergent self-aware proto-energy having no time and space can't be pinned down. We exist everywhere because we exist both as a nonspatial, indeterminate, infinite existent—a self-aware proto-energy being—and as a discrete, determinate, finite existent—a body. Thus, we exist as reality wherever our mind, our awareness, is. Others can perceive us everywhere or nowhere because human existence *is* reality. We exist everywhere as existentiality when we exist somewhere as reality, and exist nowhere as existentiality when we exist nowhere as reality. For example, when we exist unembodied—without a spirit or physical body—then to the embodied, having a physical or spirit body, we exist nowhere as reality even while we *do* exist (unembodied) as existentiality.

In practice emergent *Life*, which Philosophy with a capital-P thinks of in terms of mind or consciousness, never *doesn't* exist *as* reality because it *always* exists *as* existentiality, thus, *as* reality to itself. Molly, despite Mike in their early years having no awareness of her and therefore, to him, a nonreality of nonexistence, was a reality to herself withal, her own existent.

We can easily see our universe in these existence-as-existentiality and existence-as-reality terms. But, until now, we couldn't see All Existence because it exists solely *as* Way of Being without any empirical existents. From our perspective, All Existence is simply invisible and without existence; a nonexistent entity. This is how Philosophy with a capital-P perceives what it can't observe. Although nonexistent as existentiality, it is perceptible as reality. This very bare bones analysis needs await proper development in a later book. However, you can catch a fuller discussion than what's here in *The Story of Life* § 5:294–297.

Section 6
Way of Being

To finish out this chapter, let's consider Way of Being in a bit more detail. It's a key component even here in a book about healing your physical body because everything in All Existence, including your body, has Way of Being. It's fundamentally what anything is and the only true way to describe anything beyond its functionality.

The target of healing, for example, is Way of Being. Healing transforms your body's current Way of Being closer to emergent Way of Being, which is the Way of Being of your body at its physical conception following your emergent birth as a self-aware proto-energy being. As your body's Way of Being transforms in the Intentional healing process, the 'energies' of your body transform into the 'energy' of your body's emergent Way of Being. This necessarily transforms your body's existence and functionality as an expression of 'energy' from unhealth to health. This is the essence of physical healing. It's why we use the term 'transform' instead of 'heal.'

In this section we consider Way of Being in terms of All Existence, as self-organized, and as human.

6.1 All Existence Way of Being

Physicists will tell you that our physical universe has a normative existence, that the so-called laws of physics are the same everywhere (*SOL* § 6.1:165). This doesn't apply only to the expression of applied energy E in the natural environment, or of supra E in the supranatural environment (*SOL* § 1.2.1.2:467). It applies to all facets of integrated All Existence existing in accord with its Way of Being. At a non-aesthetic level, this means each universe's structure and operation integrates the principles—Way of Being—of All Existence. Physics, therefore, is fundamentally invariant from one universe to another as it is from galaxy to galaxy in our own universe. With our present unawareness, however, non-fundamental variations might surprise us. The recently deployed James Webb Space Telescope is surprising astronomy with such variations right now. Our experience of reality is more or less the same experience any person has anywhere in our universe and in any universe of the megaverse.

Such fundamentality of experience means that we collectively share a sense of existence *as* reality and the human place within it. Unembodied persons who experience many universes—like physical individuals traveling the globe—understand that human beings are the same in their essence everywhere. However unconsciously felt, our collective experience of existence across megaversal humanity informs our experience of existence here in our universe and on Earth. Accordingly, humanity's collective experience of existence is fundamentally a shared reality. This is partly the mechanism—not societal processes—behind the observation of communal intuition leading to multiple, independent discovery also known as simultaneous invention.

6.2 Self-organized Way of Being

Does ℒife arise preprogrammed? In a sense, it does, but it doesn't lock us in as is the case with anything 𝕃iving. A bacteria, worm, or monkey can't change *how* it is, but you can. A computer metaphor is helpful here (it doesn't imply any sort of reality, it merely helps us visualize it). We might think of Way of Being as the human operating system (os) written and pre-initialized during ℒife's emergent self-organization that boots up at process completion (phase three of conception) and runs in the central processing unit (cpu), which is our consciousness.

The operating system doesn't compile into machine code, because that would make it uneditable without a shutdown, recompile, and reboot. ℒife doesn't do that for obvious reasons. Instead, our operating system is more like a runtime interpreter with a set of libraries and such, all of which are editable at will via ℒife's *force of Intentionality* that mind mobilizes. The interpreter analyzes each line of code in context with the operating system in toto, initializes or reinitializes this or that as necessary, then interprets and executes.

Core operating system modules and subroutines are locked in terms of *how* they execute but not in terms of *what*. If it wasn't locked, we could alter our Way of Being in such a way as to make ℒife impossible and we'd irretrievably system crash—experience ℒife death, analogous to an archí dephasing—with no coming back. Emergent ℒife self-organized away from that. For example, while *mind* is a core operating system module of ℒife proto-energy 'hardware,' the *content* of mind, without which we'd be just an empty husk, is more a library of operating system 'software' that we can rewrite down to the nub until all that's left is structure.

This is why we observe in ourselves seemingly preprogrammed instincts, behaviors, needs, wants, or dispositions that Philosophy with a capital-P ascribes to our physical evolution from prehuman to human with an immutable human nature. But, in truth, these are *self-organized* traits intrinsic of Energent proto-life that self-organizes into a unique being having these traits as well as *habituated* traits arising in megaversal humanity that, in individuals, *collectively appear* intrinsic of humanity. The cool bit is that these traits are fully editable. They don't lock us into just one type of *individual* Way of Being. This is how ҢumanWay of Being both emergently self-organized and habituated traits that subconsciously edited individual Way of Being. . . resulting for us in illness, disease, aging, and death (*see* SOL § 3.3:283 for more).

6.3 Ңuman Way of Being

One doesn't feel per se the culture that permeates one's friendships, family, city, state, nation, or all human beings of Earth. Nevertheless, the Way of Being of each defines the person. Each one separately and altogether affects and in some ways governs how we think, feel, and act. For example, the more ensconced one is in a culture—mindset—the less one can think, feel, and act outside its scope of influence.

The impossibility of dissolving the Negative Collective Consciousness (NCC; CH. 1 THE NEGATIVE COLLECTIVE CONSCIOUSNESS:13) that arose in consequence of The Corruption is a case in point. Once so-called archangel Michael revealed Accountableism's fallacy (*below*; SOL § 1.4:14), the NCC stood exposed in the minds of all spirit humanity in our universe. Or, too, in breaking the four-minute mile where, despite athletes running their fastest, no one could complete a mile under four minutes until one person did, then anyone did. Both were simply mindset limitations, a subconscious unwillingness to embody what Canadian-born psychologist Albert Bandura calls self-efficacy: having a fixed versus a growth mindset (1963; 1986; 1995; 1997).

6.3.1 Accountableism, Culture, and Ultraculture

The Story of Ł ife's concept of *Accountableism* is that one is accountable to a universal moral standard—a Divine Creator: a Being or universal Truth that's necessarily imbued with infallibility thus divinity—for their behavior in thought and deed. This belief in divine accountability is Accountableism. The nature of Accountableism necessarily requires blame and the shared enforcement of the universal moral standard (Divine Will). This means living in accord with a Creator's divine—ultimate—harmlessness which *necessarily is harm*. Until the Big Healing, Accountableism was perforce our universal culture, which is *Ultraculture* (SOL § 4.1:291).

Ultraculture is so global that it's subliminal. Its effect on the individual is limited to their sense of humanity, of what it means to be themself in human terms. Like the NCC, it's locally weak yet globally strong. One might think they feel human simply on account of being born, raised, and existing amongst humans as a human. Yet, a person born and self-raised in isolation—however animalistic, noncognitive, or mentally disabled they may appear to be—nevertheless responds intrinsically humanly which, absent brain damage, is evident upon recovery. One can't humanize a chimp. But a human raised by chimps who thinks he or she is a chimp remains human, hence, humanizable out of the chimp's milieu.

The problem in feral child cases in the context of The Corruption and subpar mind–brain integration is that, once one isolates from the human milieu, the brain repurposes to its environment. Mind–brain integration then degrades further in a self-reinforcing cycle. Such a person's spirit self remains fully, experientially human having Ꜧuman Way of Being. But their physical embodiment, their 'avatar' in the physical world, is out of the loop. Their physically instantiated mind habituates to their environment.

An individual's experience with their own individual culture is fully active, not passive, despite larger cultures negligibly contributing to it. One's experience with culture farther from own-self is an active–passive matrix that becomes more passive and less active the farther from own-self it gets. Experiencing a universal culture is fully passive despite own-self negligibly contributing to it. Humans experience the *reality* of Ꜧuman Way of Being through their own individual Way of Being and feel the *experience* of Ꜧuman Way of Being just as universal humanity collectively embodies in universal culture. Individuals passively experience the reality of humanity collectively in its nonautonomy, existence, and Intentionality via the Way of Being effect on Ultraculture that we've just described. Let's consider these collective experiences.

6.3.2 Way of Being of the Physical Body

Like everything, our body has Way of Being: *emergent* Way of Being and *attributive* Way of Being (CH. 7 § 1.1.1:164). Your attributive Way of Being arises in your subconscious–conscious mind as a habituated response to encountered 'energy.' It then becomes your physical body's own attributive Way of Being. This is because the Intentional machine that's your proto-energy self ever Intentionalizing 'energy' into your body stamps it over—negates—your body's emergent Way of Being.

6.3.3 Emergent Way of Being

For Philosophy with a capital-P, about the only agreed-upon definition of life is that entities possessing it exhibit certain characteristics that sum up to a state of being that's called alive. These include cellular organization and metabolism in a homeostatic environment that shows growth, adaptation, stimuli response, and reproductive ability (SOL § 1.1:532). But these functions define only a state of Living; such automata don't add up to having Life. It might seem like it does materially (bodily). But it doesn't with mind—psyche—for the straightforward reason that biology is Living matter and mind isn't. Even taking the position that mind arises in biology, we're still left with mind being not-biology—at least in terms of cellular automata, a specific enzymatic, hormonal, or cellular mechanism in and of itself being thinking, feeling, intuition . . . the whole gamut of mind experience—but an apparent emergent property sans physicality.

Science reckons biology as alive with certain caveats. If we imbue that with Life, however, we lose the nonconscious distinction with consciousness, the ineffable emergent *being* having Life where we distinguish Life from lowercase-l life as uniquely human versus Living from lowercase-l living as uniquely nonhuman. Then, what does it mean to *have* Life versus Living? We answer this by comprehending what it means to be human, since humanness is the sum total essence of consciousness as personness.

6.3.4 Emergence of Life

Life is unique to All Existence, not just to our (much less any) universe. It doesn't arise in evolutionary biology as does Living. Life is human; human is Life. In the process chain of emergence, Life is what emergently births albeit not as a trait or property. It self-organizes as a particular Way of Being that is consciousness as personness, humanness—an eternal, self-existent being. It's an existent of humanness in terms of functionality (consciousness) and singularity (personness) of being. As noted, after Life spontaneously birthed as the first two emergent persons (Mike and Molly), it arises afterward only from pairwise human Intentionality. That is to say, it isn't random nor sperm-meets-egg biology. Life arises in three contexts because a person exists simultaneously in one, two, or three states of being: unembodied (everyone), spirit-embodied (spirit-born and physical-born), and physical-embodied (physical-born).

In this book, we only deal with physical embodiment (you can read about unembodiment and spirit-embodiment in SOL § 1.2.1:247). You initially experience ℒife physically embodied in the objective, somatic natural environment of our universe through an *objective body*. In this mode of ℒife, your body is a biological existent that you, a self-aware proto-energy being, integrate. That means your body is a reality in its own right with its own processes, needs, and intrinsic behaviors.

You also experience ℒife spirit embodied in the supranatural environment of our universe through a *subjective body*. While we can materially affect our physical body, we can't change it wholesale as we can our spirit body in the spirit mode of ℒife. This is because the physical body operates in accord with absolute biological parameters. If we obviate those, the body loses sustainment. You, like most, may think of the physical mode of ℒife as regular life, the only *real* life. Intrinsically, this physical state of being is more albeit not anywhere near as limited as it appears today. Educable awareness rectifies our ignorance of our physical embodiment. Accordingly, physical life is not less than—meaning base, unsacred—than spirit life.

Although there's an obvious functional difference between these three contexts of being, unembodiment isn't intrinsically better, more enlightened, more spiritual, or closer to the Divine than embodiment. A physical-born person who, after death, chooses to live unembodied isn't any different from, say, a Japan-born person emigrating to America to 'disembody' their Japanism and embody Americanism. In each case, they're the same person only in a different context. Because you aren't your body. You are mind.

Section 7
Conclusion to Chapter 2

This chapter is rather a heavy-duty affair. It introduces you to a host of new concepts regarding the origin and function of our human existence and the larger milieu in which you experience life. Let's sum it up.

All Existence is 'all there infinitely is.' It exists not like outer space that we can observe and fly spaceships through to other planets and maybe one day to galaxies, but *as* Way of Being. Its fundamental aspect *is* Energent–prime, which fundamental essence is proto-energy, which fundamental expression is *enérgeia*. The Energent proto-energy of our universe *is* Energent–prime proto-energy. It suffuses not only All Existence but every crumb and scrap of our own (and every) universe, including your physical body.

Human ℒife is an emergent aspect of Energent proto-life, itself an emergent property of All Existence. Humanity, which is to say, ℒife, emergently birthed pairwise in an unembodied state close to 800 billion years ago. For convenience, we call these very first two humans Mike and Molly. Their emergent birth was *spontaneous*. You emergently birthed as one aspect of pairwise ꞪHuman Way of Being, which embodiments Mike and Molly established as male–female and collective humanity *habituated* as individual Way of Being. Your emergent birth was not spontaneous like Mike and Molly's but *triggered* by pairwise humans—your parents.

Your physical body physically conceives as an *objective* aspect of your emergent birth 'in' Energent proto-life, which itself is an emergent, ℒife-precursor property of *non-self-aware* All Existence. Your spirit body manifests as a *subjective* property of your self-aware proto-energy self. Altogether, your integrated physical and spirit bodies render you a *physicospirit* person who simultaneously exists and interacts with the natural (physical) environment and the supranatural (spirit) environment. Your existence in the universe is wholistic, unlimited, infinite (indeterminate). You are limited only by your beliefs and mindset.

Mind–brain integration along with mind–body integration effectively means your physical body is literally a manifestation, or instantiation, of mind that comports with your beliefs and mindset. For example, if you subconsciously believe your physical body is naught but animal and subject to—a victim of—natural biological processes, then your Intentional mind makes it so. If you don't, then it isn't.

Your psyche (consciousness) exists discretely 'in' Energent proto-life (EPL), yet it's as infinite as All Existence in that, through awareness, it's not limited by time and space. This means you can be *everywhere* you want to be 'in' All Existence in accord with your EPL-intrinsic nondimensionality and your exerted awareness yet, at the same time, *nowhere* 'in' All Existence. This is a sharp philosophical point. You can find a deeper discussion on it in *The Story of ℒife* § 5:294–297.

Way of Being is the 'how' something is at its most fundamental. Like All Existence and our universe, ꞪHuman has Way of Being and you, the individual, have individual Way of Being. Your body has emergent—original—Way of Being as well as attributive—mind-developed—Way of Being. The latter is what you're transforming to the former when you (or a healer) exert Intentional healing on your body.

Comprehending the topics covered in this chapter will greatly help you understand and exert Intentional healing, although a healer can heal you regardless (cf. CH. 8 § 2.1:172). Toward that end, we more fully discuss mind in the next chapter.

3

The Bell of the Mind

This chapter combines some of *The Story of Life*'s Chapter 26 on the mind with newly energy-tested information about the subconscious. The reason for this chapter and Chapter 2 is that all of your physical body health issues, including the effects of aging, arise in your mind not your body. You can't effectively heal yourself without understanding how your mind works with respect to your body. Although a healer can heal you, your mind will resist it to varying degrees. This drags out the healing process or negates it altogether. Not everybody wants to master self-healing; you might prefer a healer do the work. But if you want to heal yourself (plus, perhaps, others) then everything in this book is critical, need-to-know information. Let's begin with an overview of mind.

Section 1
The Nature of Mind

We tend to think our phenomenal environment defines absolute reality. That's a distraction. Our mind is the real environment in which we exist because that's where we *experience* phenomenal—natural, physical—reality, although that's only one aspect of an individual's overall reality. When we think of mind as infinite—indeterminate—as space, yet the physicospirit universe as existentially static where mind is functionally dynamic, we see that, unlike a universe, the very nature of mind is always in flux. After all, mind creates universe. The phenomenal universe is a real extension of mind because we can mold it to our will like a universe builder or the way universal humanity Intentionalized the Negative Collective Consciousness (dissolved October 13, 2017).

We live consciously mired in phenomenal reality severed from the fullness of ℒife and unable to imagine it beyond our physical embodiment. We build relationships, societies, and knowledge rooted only in what our bodies can sense. We interact with others without regard for our physicospirit reality, boxing ourselves into the here and now of physical survival. We live not *like* animals but *as* animals. Science then concludes we're just the cleverest of the kind. But we're not animals. Though we oft think our body is literally *us*, the person we are, it's only an 'avatar,' an embodiment. We blithely discount mind as a mystery of brain the way religion discounts reality as a mystery of faith and science discounts (especially quantum) existence as a mystery of creation.

If you sit down, close your eyes . . . just let your thoughts roam, you tend to lose track of your physical environment till it has no bearing on what's happening in your mind. You could, for example, genuinely be on Saturn. Until you open your eyes. The physical environment materially affects your body but not your mind, which experiences what your physical body encounters just as it does what your spirit body encounters. And, too, mind encounters itself. It experiences what it conjures. When you're imagining yourself on Saturn, you're experiencing Saturn as your mind creates it. Its true physical reality is immaterial. For mind, experience *is* reality. People imagining themselves on a peaceful tropical beach open their eyes not having *imagined* themselves refreshed, calmed, or relaxed but authentically feeling, *experiencing*, it. This chapter describes mind with respect to its nature and experience because that's our true reality. It's what we actually experience, not phenomenality which we only encounter (*sol* § 1.1.1:362). Mind's emergent nature is that it constitutes of those aspects traditionally termed subconscious and conscious. Mind's undulant experience—rising and falling in awareness and response—is literally all there is to the person. You are what you experience, not what you encounter.

Mind is different from psyche which, traditionally, is understood as consciousness. It's an *expression* of psyche but not psyche itself. You as a ℘erson, as ℌuman, aren't your mind in the way humanity has customarily encountered it but ℒife itself. In essence, you are *emergent self-aware proto-energy* (*Fig. 3.1, left*). At its most fundamental, ℒife is self-aware

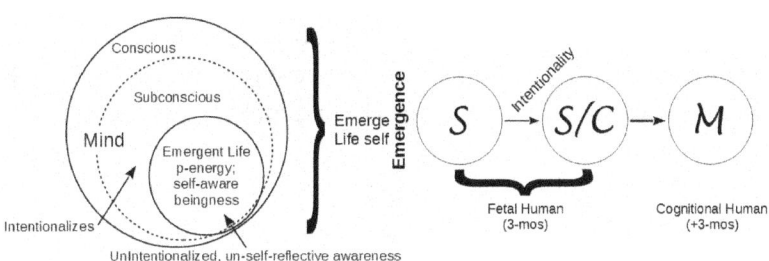

Fig. 3.1. Left, schematic: wholistic, emergent ℒife self that Intentionalizes mind. Energent–prime and proto-energy is logically (⇔) equivalent to consciousness/psyche and the self-aware proto-energy self. *Right*, emergent ℒife self (S) emergently (spontaneously) Intentionalizes subconscious–conscious mind (S/C) from which the 3-month fetal human transitions to 3-month-plus cognitional human (M).

but not self-reflective. The latter is mind's job, which your ℒife self (your self-aware beingness) Intentionalizes into reality soon after emergent birth as your means to encounter and experience 'energy' outside your being (*Fig. 3.1, right*). We therefore necessarily distinguish between self-aware beingness and mind, where self-aware beingness is emergent proto-energy/psyche—consciousness—though not exactly. We *are* the former but express wholistically *as* the latter via its conscious and subconscious aspects.

A person emergently—spontaneously—Intentionalizes their own subconscious–conscious from their self-aware proto-energy self as an aspect of fundamental Way of Being within about three months of emergent birth. In practical terms, this means about three months after physical or spirit conception. We identify the person up to this approximately 3-month point as *fetal human* who is unaware of his or her existence, reality, and environment but *is* self-aware.

It's important to note that ℒ*ife is fully human from emergent birth*. The fetal human isn't less than or pre-human—lacking Ꜧuman Way of Being—just because he or she is unaware of their existence in reality and hasn't yet Intentionalized their mind interface. On the contrary, the self-aware person is complete in all respects at the very instant of emergent birth having self-aware beingness and absolute autonomy (Ꜧuman Way of Being; cf. ABORTION *SOL* § 2.2:410). We identify the post-fetal person as *cognitional* human, where cognitional isn't a physiological result but a mind-awareness result.

Mind is like a universe's dual (natural–supranatural) environment in the context of one's emergent ℒife self, which itself is like All Existence. For example, a builder Intentionalizes a universe 'out of' proto-energy to therein experience external-to-mind phenomenal reality—All Existence being its own kind of 'phenomenality'—via the interface of embodiment. Similarly, a person's subconscious Intentionalizes states of being and states of awareness as a foundation upon which conscious mind experiences external-to-subconscious-mind reality. The subconscious Intentionalizes an aspect of itself to have awareness of external-to-mind 'energies.' This is the conscious mind. Wholistic mind experiences its environment as awareness of 'energy' conceptually similar to how a bat has environmental awareness via echolocation. Mind is the only Intentional cause—a source that produces a result—in emergent All Existence.

It's impossible to think of mind in terms of cognition. Mind is protoenergy that experiences reality as awareness. It's so fast and wholistic it defies real description with a vocabulary limited by our inurement to comprehending everything solely in terms of biochemistry where cognitional brain is consciousness. To understand the conscious and subconscious, we need develop a wholistic awareness of mind. This means comprehending it in its natural habitat of proto-energy that's emergently self-aware. We term this wholistic understanding *experience of mind*, to which we now turn.

Section 2
Experience of Mind

2.1 Subconscious–conscious Mind

Our subconscious is who we are. It's our who-ness (SOL § 2.1.1.1:368). It constitutes about 99.996% of wholistic mind despite conventional notions that mind is 5–10% visible (conscious) iceberg with 90–95% hidden subsurface. The subconscious is deductive. Its awareness—not reasoning—moves from the general to the particular, from premise to specifics. This is opposite the inductive nature of conscious mind (SOL § 2.2:395). But keep cognizant that subconscious doesn't engage in thinking–feeling, i.e., Thought. That's conscious mind's Way of Being (SOL § 2.2.1.1:234). Subconscious simply has *awareness* of everything that conscious mind encounters. Conscious mind operates vis-à-vis subconscious the way brain operates vis-à-vis wholistic Life mind (SOL § 2.1:276).

We're used to thinking our conscious mind is our conscious*ness*, who we are. But that's an inaccurate observation born of our inability to perceive physicospirit reality. All of our thinking–feeling originates as wholistic states of being (SOB) and states of awareness (SOA) in the subconscious that Intentionalizes infinite SOB and SOA to the conscious mind where we parse them as Thought. Subconscious awareness is not simply too fast for our brain to operate on. Its mode of awareness is incompatible with the brain's functionality of cognition, too. It thus requires transliteration from one environment to the other. This is what *The Story of Life* calls mind–brain integration.

The bottom line here is that *you are only partly your conscious mind*, which is the environment of your experience, inner voice, and thinking–feeling. *You are far more your subconscious*, which is the environment of your awareness, ideas, drive, ambition, and Way of Being. Mike and Molly discovered that mind–brain integration patterns itself on the nature of emergent Life mind (SOL § 2.1.5:313). Conscious mind transliterates subconscious awareness to conscious cognitional beingness just as brain transliterates Life mind's awareness into its cognitive beingness (SOL § 1.2.2.4:257; SOL § 2.6:402). The cognitional beingness we're talking about here isn't the cognitive *mental process* of knowing as with brain (SOL § 2.1:276), but "that which *comes to be known*," not as a product of a mental process but of *awareness* (*American*, s.v. 2 'cognition,' *ia*). Conscious awareness differs from subconscious awareness in that conscious mind is awareness of infinite segmented states of being and states of awareness whereas subconscious awareness is that of an individual's wholistic state of being and state of awareness.

Your proto-energy self is emergently self-aware. It's not the same thing as subconscious–conscious. The fundament of Ƕuman is self-aware proto-energy. You are pure awareness. There is no thinking, feeling, or self-reflection in that. There's only awareness that forms a state of being and state of awareness. It is self-aware but not cognitive. It's an emergent Life being that's *aware* of itself and reality, aware of its awareness, and aware that it's aware of its awareness, but it doesn't self-reflect (SOL § 1.2.2.1:253). Conscious mind does the self-analysis because it transliterates wholistic, subconscious state of being and state of awareness into small, segmented states of being and states of awareness that are operable. It's similar to reducing a problem unsolvable in its entirety to many small, solvable ones.

This means conscious mind cognizes the singular, wholistic state of being and state of awareness that is subconscious as its many constituent SOB–SOA aspects such that it can analyze, self-reflect upon, think–feel about, and mix and match them. Think of subconscious like an infinite reservoir from which conscious mind is constantly sipping, tasting, experiencing, interpreting, thinking–feeling, and so forth its full flavor. Not simply that of the sip, but of the entire reservoir that's embodied in the individual sip. Each sip constitutes a *focal awareness* in the context of *wholistic awareness*. Subconscious–conscious *is* wholistic mind.

Conscious mind is the retarded—slowed-down—*aspect* of subconscious. It's not a separate mind or a version of the subconscious. It's an aspect of self experiencing subconscious awareness of external-to-mind 'energies.' This makes it discriminatory as a function of its Way of Being between 'energies' as a means to comprehend them whereas subconscious has awareness of *all* 'energies.' From conscious mind's discriminatory Way of Being arises its analytical Way of Being that constitutes Thought, which we're used to as the foundational capabilities of mind. Subconscious has awareness of all that conscious mind encounters. To express its discriminatory Way of Being, conscious mind Intentionalizes with an inductive Way of Being. This means reasoning from detailed facts to general principles, from specifics to a premise. In other words, rather than experiencing a *wholistic* awareness of its environment the way subconscious has awareness, it segments it into discrete *experiences* of awareness. Where subconscious doesn't act on any particular state of being and state of awareness associated with some discrete experience of awareness but rather has individual, discrete states of being and states of awareness as a wholistic awareness, conscious mind acts on *each* discrete experience of awareness it encounters. This *acting* is what constitutes Thought (thinking–feeling).

Because subconscious–conscious are altogether mind, then what conscious mind encounters—its awareness of it, how it experiences it—is all as intimately known to subconscious as it is to conscious mind. But subconscious doesn't actually *experience* external-to-mind reality, it only has *awareness* of what's experienced by conscious mind. This means that subconscious forms its own state of being and state of awareness of each experience of which conscious mind is aware. Its awareness of conscious mind's experience may or may not differ from conscious mind's own awareness because, while conscious mind is in practice *a part of* its (inclusive of external-to-mind) environment, subconscious is not. It has no interaction *with*, only awareness *of*, conscious mind's environment.

A human being is a person of singular SOB–SOA. There are no internal contradictions between how one experiences external-to-mind reality and own-self as well as conscious experiences relative to own-self. Because both aspects of mind constitute a singular being and dichotomies arise between subconscious awareness and conscious experience, then a *reconciliation* between awareness and experience is necessary for a singular being to have a singular state of being and state of awareness. Otherwise, such dichotomies result in internal contradiction that eventually give rise to experiences like Post-traumatic Stress Disorder (PTSD).

Ideally, subconscious should be as consciously accessible as what we'd normally consider conscious awareness. The Corruption caused us to Intentionalize the Negative Collective Consciousness. This brought about a generalized negative thinking–feeling and produced in our lack of awareness a dysfunction in the psyche not to mention of our universe generally (this is amenable as a result of so-called archangel Michael and Lucifer's Reconciliation; CH. 7 § 1.1:163; CH. 8 § 1:169; *TBH* CH. 4; *SOL* § 4.2:379; *SOL* § 4.2.1.4:382). By energy testing, for example, you develop greater awareness of subconscious because you access different aspects of 'mind energy' according to how you test. Conscious mind develops exquisite sensitivity not only to ambient 'energy' but to that of subconscious as well. In this way, a person can develop functional awareness of subconscious and no longer be in the dark regarding the origin of their thinking–feeling nor endure experiences likened to so-called self-sabotage.

Because The Corruption interfered with mindset and, ultimately, mind–brain integration—transliteration—we experience a mental blindness concomitant with a structural limitation in the brain that limits awareness and how much of mind can integrate brain at any given moment (*SOL* § 1.2.2.5:261). The practical result is that we're cut off from the fullness of *L*ife and unable to experience most of our own states of awareness. This isn't a permanent condition, however. Mina's been rectifying it since the October 13, 2017 Big Healing and, with that, our ever-plastic brain restores the necessary neural structure long ago discarded.

2.1.1 Subconscious and Mind–body Integration

Recall that subconscious–conscious integrates brain while subconscious as an aspect of emergent self integrates body. Here, we describe mind–body integration in terms of the 'energy' of emergent self. This 'energy' integrates each bonded archí pair of the body. It establishes the 'energy' of complex archí structures leading to molecules that result in DNA and RNA thus the body's biochemistry and biofunctionality. In the context of emergent Way of Being (versus attributive Way of Being), mind–body integration is properly understood as *awareness*-body integration—we stick with familiar mind–body nomenclature for clarity—and that's all: no conscious, no subconscious, only awareness. This means your body literally forms out of the 'energy' of emergent self in the process of your self-aware proto-energy self—your emergent self, i.e., wholistic awareness—integrating your two-going-on-four embryonic cells through to body death.

Subconscious–conscious as wholistic mind are *aspects of awareness* of your self-aware proto-energy self. Conscious awareness is like the 'skin' of your emergent self in the context of Energent proto-life that experiences every nuance of 'energy' external to own-self the way your body's skin experiences every nuance of the physical environment external to the body. To carry this analogy a bit further, subconscious awareness is like the nerves in the skin and tissue interacting with the skin's interaction with the environment to fire off nerve impulses—action potentials—having no awareness of the nature of the skin–environment interaction. Subconscious thusly Intentionalizes the 'energy' that conscious awareness encounters having no awareness of the nature of the conscious/external-to-mind interaction.

For example, you bump your knee. Subconscious exerts an Intentional response analogous to neural impulses arising in your skin that, in accord with subconscious 'belief'—attributive habits—manifests in your knee as pain, bruising, damage, maybe the rise of a chronic condition. Your body is a neural machine analogous to your proto-energy self as an Intentional machine. You train subconscious Intentional reactions to remove attributive habits damaging your body similar to training your body's neural reactions to remove, say, unhelpful (potentially damaging) reflexes.

Your physical body via mind–body (awareness–body) integration is the 'skin' of wholistic awareness (subconscious–conscious) in the physical context as your spirit body is its 'skin' in the spirit context. Your properly integrated physical body is not one bit different from your spirit body except for its matter limitations that your spirit body, manifested of supramatter, doesn't have. Your body is an *extension* of subconscious (emergent self). They are one and the same. Hence, the 'energy' of mind–body integration is the 'energy' of emergent self. Mind–body integration is literally pure awareness of the physical environment. Accordingly, the 'energy' of your body is the 'energy' of integration, which is the 'energy' of awareness, which is emergent proto-life, which expression is 𝓛ife force—self-aware proto-energy encapsulating emergent Way of Being—emanating from the self-aware proto-energy person, i.e., your emergent self.

2.1.2 What is Subconscious 'Belief'

Mind lives in whatever reality it determines is real. Your sense of reality arises altogether in subconscious–conscious, which is to say, wholistic mind. No matter where it is or what it's doing, mind chooses how the body and environment manifest. Don't be fooled by the evidence of matter. That, because it feels more solid and real than Thought then matter is your definitive reality. That because, say, you've been diagnosed with cancer, which you comprehend as a material reality, then that defines your physical state of being. Mind transcends matter because it's an Intentionalized aspect of self. In the context of our universe, matter arises in Energent proto-energy, which itself responds to the Intentionality of your emergent proto-energy self, the very *you* that is you. Accordingly, matter responds to the Intentionality of mind. You therefore choose your body's manifestation because you are an Intentional being, not an animal. You are Ꮧuman. No one can change your mind to create your reality but you. Your body only ever manifests *your* reality. If you don't like your reality (say, cancer), you can learn how to change it.

Subconscious 'belief' is what mind accepts as real. Attributive habit is the 'energy' of which subconscious is aware plus Intentionalized damage that mind–body integrates; thus, its reality. Hence, 'belief' is an aspect of awareness. We typeset belief in single quotes to indicate it's not belief in its traditional definition as some cognitive content or a state or habit of mind that's held as true. 'Belief' as we use it here means *your proto-energy self's 'energy' awareness that may or may not Intentionalize*. Recall that subconscious doesn't think in the way we imagine conscious mind thinking. It doesn't scheme or punish or thwart you; subconscious self-sabotage is a mistaken assumption. It doesn't *know* or *feel* things. It just *does* things. It simply experiences external-to-self 'energy' and responds to that 'energy' in terms of its own 'energy' awareness in the same conceptual way that nerve endings respond to stimulus, although subconscious awareness is much more than nerve ending stimulus. This 'energy' awareness is what people think of as subconscious belief.

Why does subconscious experience 'energy' in the way that it does, say, in contradiction to conscious Thought? For example, you encounter 'energy' in the world which subconscious interprets—experiences—as your body being frail and subject to damage and death that your conscious mind may repudiate. Why does subconscious ignore conscious mind to experience 'energy' in that way and embrace it as real? Why does that 'energy' then become the 'energy' of emergent self, which Intentionalizes into your body? We answer each question in turn.

2.1.2.1 Why Does Subconscious Experience 'Energy' as It Does?

Subconscious *vibes* with the 'energy' it encounters—for example, 'energy' of damage and death as the physical human reality. By vibe, we mean that subconscious has awareness of external-to-self 'energy' as though *its own*. From its perspective—how it experiences 'energy'—external 'energy' *is* your self-aware proto-energy self's own 'energy.' There is no distinction between external-to-self 'energy' and own-self 'energy.' This is analogous to nerve endings encountering stimulus—'energy'—as if of the body. The reason that subconscious vibes with such 'energy' is because *it has no awareness of the 'energy' of ℒife force* (*below*). It therefore has no other 'energy' to vibe with. Such external-to-self 'energy' is the only game in town. Why would this be so? The reason is The Corruption. Let's explain.

Like All Existence, The Corruption can only be described *as* Way of Being. Specifically, it is Intentionalized Way of Being. As it's Intentionalized, it is 'mind energy.' This means it's uniquely human, i.e., ℒife. Any Way of Being outside of fundamental existence—All Existence, Energent proto-life, and ℒife, each of which constitutes of *emergent* Way of Being in context—arises in human Intentionality. For example, Mina Intentionalized the Way of Being of everything in our universe as its creation process, excluding ℒife which emergently births. Therefore, other persons necessarily Intentionalized all other Ways of Being in our universe... The Corruption to cite the first significant instance, and the Negative Collective Consciousness to cite the second.

'Mind energy,' which a person Intentionalizes, interacts with Energent proto-energy that suffuses our universe. Proto-energy responds to Intentionalized 'mind energy.' This is the uniqueness of ℒife. It's why we say that any external-to-self-encounter to which subconscious responds—experiences—*is* 'energy.' Accordingly, we fundamentally define The Corruption *as* 'energy,' which *is* 'mind energy' embodying a certain Thought in toto constituting a particular Way of Being. *The Story of ℒife* explains this *as* Accountableism principally embodied in altruism. We don't describe The Corruption's process and methodology here (*see* SOL § 2:367), but its 'energy' drenches all human 'energy' in our universe.

This human 'energy' does not include ℒife force, however. Recall that ℒife force is the individual human person's emergent proto-energy—the 'energy' that is you—incorporating emergent Way of Being. These are emergent properties of the person, not Intentionalized by another person but emergently birthing 'in' Energent proto-life. ℒife force, uniquely representing the person's emergent proto-energy and emergent Way of Being, is an *internal reality*. It is *individual*. It does not Intentionalize into a person nor their physical body. It simply *is*. With respect to mind integrating body, ℒife force suffuses body because body *is* mind. Hence, the 'energy' of body *is* the 'energy' of Life force, *the* fundamental expression of the self-aware proto-energy self—*you*.

On the other hand, all other 'energy' that one encounters in existence is external to the person and, therefore, an *external reality*. Ordinarily, one's internal reality would be fundamental and external reality secondary. The Corruption reversed this by Intentionalizing a barrier, so to speak, between mind and physicospirit reality. In consequence, physical humanity lost its awareness of the 'energy' of Life force. This means that our self-aware proto-energy self—the fundamental aspect of what we are as beings having Life—*has no awareness of the 'energy' of Life force*. A person doesn't know what that 'energy' is; doesn't know how it feels.

For example, consider subconscious a sheet of paper, the 'energy' of damage—attributive habit—an alpha particle, and Life force gamma radiation. Paper stops—interacts with thus has 'awareness' of—alpha particles but gamma rays pass through; paper has no awareness of it. Life force suffuses subconscious but it has no awareness of its 'energy,' only the 'energy' of attributive habit. *That* 'energy' *is* subconscious 'energy' thus, via mind–body integration, the 'energy' of body. Our experience of it is so minuscule as to be effectively nonexistent. Hence, the only 'energy' we *do* experience is the 'energy' of The Corruption. In our physical body context, this means our subconscious experiences this 'energy'—that our physical body is frail and aging inevitably toward death—as what's fundamentally real.

This arose in our loss of awareness of human physicospirit reality caused by the loss of full mind–brain integration that the Intentionality of The Corruption encapsulated. This is why the physical-born—you and me—have until now had no awareness of the 'energy' of Life force. Physical humanity has been addicted to the mindset of physical frailty as our one and only reality of physical existence. Awareness shows us there's a choice. It shows us our unlimited possibilities, immediately bringing our body transformation. We then make an Intentional choice, whatever it may be.

Our physical body being subject to the vagaries of physical existence is a *false premise* because we believe we have no choice in that it's the way we are, that it's our foundational Way of Being, an *objective* fact. But it's a *subjective* reality. Therefore, the premise is false. As soon as we have awareness that reality is *our* choice, and we make that choice, then it's no longer a false premise but our *true premise* because we've made it so.

This means that your body being frail and subject to the harsh realities of biology is not, in and of itself, a false premise nor a false reality. It's a false premise only because humanity believes it to be an objective fact when it's merely subjective reality. It's your *true* premise and reality because your subconscious, in its unawareness of your physicospirit reality, accepted it, Intentionalized it, and lives with it. If you change your choice, you change what you now take for the false premise that you *can* Intentionally heal your body to your true premise and, thereby, change what you now take for the true premise that you *cannot* Intentionally heal your body to your false premise.

An analogy for how each of us created our physical body as it is today is a *glamour*. This is a term for a spirit person changing how their spirit body looks or how their voice sounds (SOL § 2.1.5.4.4:318). They can do this because Intentional mind is the source of all manifestation, physical or spirit. Spirit persons *consciously* choose how they want to manifest the appearance of their spirit body to others and invest their choice with Intentionality (pain and suffering can do this subconsciously instead, such as a child remaining the same age as an unhealed trauma). And so they appear.

Similarly, physical persons *subconsciously* Intentionalize a reality onto their physical body, say, that the body can be damaged and die. And so they appear. Subconscious determines how one's physical body operates, appears, and sounds because humans are Intentional beings. Subconscious 'belief' is, effectively, a physical glamour. Once one *Intentionally chooses* to remove that glamour, then one's body *instantly is* as emergent Way of Being *is*; you have chosen to physically embody *as* emergent Way of Being.

Intentionalized proto-energy suffuses all matter in the natural (physical) environment. It accordingly affects all matter (e.g., animal bodies) with the exception of the human body which integrates mind. Your body is thereby a literal extension of mind unlike any other Living entity. Such Intentionalized proto-energy only affects the human body when subconscious, experiencing that 'energy,' Intentionalizes it into the body as we've described. Subconscious 'belief' that human bodies are subject to damage and death just like animal bodies is an Intentionality with which subconscious vibes because, until the October 13, 2017 Reconciliation, the 'energy' of The Corruption was the most powerful Intentional 'energy' in our universe that even now negates our body's emergent Way of Being.

The reason for this lies in universal humanity—spirit-born and physical-born—accepting it as real. For the spirit-born, it resulted in a society of Accountableism with its own problems for them. For the physical-born, it resulted in a society of physicospirit ignorance embodying Accountableism where physical frailty was all that was real. Absent full mind–brain integration and awareness of our physicospirit existence, this reality made primary the Intentionalized 'energy' of The Corruption as our principle awareness of 'energy' by way of degrading our awareness of the 'energy' of Ƕuman emergent Way of Being. This provoked all the problems miring physical humanity including chronic disease, injury, and death.

Matter only exists as mind Intentionalizes it. Mina Intentionalized our universe and its matter–supramatter environments. But you, and you alone, Intentionalize the 'universe' of your physical body's matter.

2.1.2.2 Why Does the 'Energy' of The Corruption Become the 'Energy' of Subconscious?

The 'energy' of The Corruption replaced the 'energy' of emergent Way of Being—an aspect of ℒife force—in our subconscious because the 'energy' of physical frailty is so much stronger than ℒife force. Why? Because the 'energy' of The Corruption (from which subconscious 'belief' in physical frailty arises) is Intentionalized 'energy' which, owing to vast universal humanity's subconscious 'belief' in its primacy, is far stronger and more prevalent in the individual than the non-Intentionalized 'energy' of emergent Way of Being. The reason is our absolute autonomy as emergent beings. Existence is what we make it. Reality is what we accept as real. The 'energy' that subconscious principally experiences is therefore the 'energy' of that reality. Accordingly, the 'energy' of emergent Way of Being is not real to our subconscious. Being not real, humanity subconsciously disregards it. Awareness of it degraded to dribs and drabs. Wherefore, the 'energy' that *is* subconscious 'belief' is the 'energy' it accepts and, consequently, the 'energy' with which it vibes.

Thus, we have no awareness in our self-aware proto-energy self of the 'energy' of ℒife force. Absent this awareness, subconscious simply vibes with the prevalent human 'energy' of our universe which, in our physical case, is the Intentionalized 'energy' that *is* the Way of Being of the body's frailty. Of course, subconscious in accord with emergent Way of Being then *integrates* this 'energy' with your physical body via subconscious mind–body integration. Subconscious, however, doesn't *Intentionalize* the 'energy' of ℒife force—emergent proto-energy incorporating emergent Way of Being—into your body. It simply *experiences* it as an aspect of emergent you. From conception, your body *is* emergent Way of Being; the 'energy' that *is* the matter–Energy of your body *is* the 'energy' of emergent Way of Being.

Absent the 'energy' of The Corruption Intentionalizing into your body like a new floor over an existing floor, your body naturally *is* the 'energy' of emergent Way of Being. Your physical body manifests that 'energy' because it is mind–body integrated. However, external-to-self 'energy,' which subconscious encounters, *does* Intentionalize. If it's strong enough to Intentionalize then, ipso facto, it is subconscious 'belief.' If it's not strong enough to Intentionalize then it's not 'belief.'

This process gives rise to *attributive Way of Being*, the subconscious Way of Being that's not emergent Way of Being. It's why subconscious does what conscious mind rejects. In humanity's present condition given The Corruption and 50,000 years of history since humans first integrated proto-human bodies on Earth, conscious mind fully embraces the frailty of the body from the moment subconscious emergently Intentionalizes into existence as described in CH. 3 § 1:95. This is the case even when we consciously don't want it, reject it, and believe we can avoid it.

The reason for this dichotomy is that conscious mind is not Intentional like subconscious, though both are aspects of emergent self. It's only Intentional when we exert conscious Thought as 'mind energy' that rises to subconscious Thought such that subconscious gets habituated (trained) to experience the 'energy' of that conscious Thought. This is conscious Intentionality. It's how one reorients subconscious, thus emergent self, to reflect conscious belief (in the traditional sense of that word and in the sense of removing so-called subconscious self-sabotage) and thereby remove the attributive Way of Being that's causing one's body to malfunction.

Damage doesn't exist in emergent Way of Being. In the context of the physical body, emergent Way of Being is its blueprint. Damage is not part of that blueprint. If that blueprint is in force—not overwhelmed by attributive Way of Being—then damage can't exist. Emergent Way of Being is always in force because it suffuses your emergent proto-energy, your body's ᴸife force, the you that is you. But Intentionalized attributive Way of Being is stronger than emergent Way of Being because the latter is *not* Intentionalized, it just *is* as incorporated in our emergent proto-energy. Attributive Way of Being, on the other hand, being Intentionality, necessarily *changes* proto-energy (that's always suffusing your body as it does all matter in the natural environment) in accord with Intentional Thought. Intentionalized attributive Way of Being is changing the whole makeup of the Energent proto-energy suffusing your body. It becomes Intentionalized by the attributive 'energy' of damage. It thusly *is* the 'energy' of damage. This is opposite the 'energy' of your unIntentionalized emergent Way of Being that merely suffuses emergent proto-energy, which is necessarily the 'energy' of no-damage. In this environment, emergent

Way of Being barely affects your body, exerting about 0.056% of what's normative. Thus, your body operates with minimal ℒife force therefore minimal natural healing.

With awareness comes choice. Choose to remove the block—stop Intentionalizing attributive Way of Being—and the 'energy' of the body 'instantly' *is* emergent proto-energy suffusing emergent Way of Being. The body then 'instantly' transforms from manifesting attributive Way of Being (damage) to manifesting emergent Way of Being (no-damage). In practical terms, this means your body 'instantly' transforms from damage to no-damage. Take note that 'instantly' in this context of *full awareness of all we've discussed* means from a picosecond to up to about 12 hours. Without such full awareness, your body transforms slower but nevertheless heals.

2.2 Conscious Awareness of Subconscious

An individual ideally has full awareness of their mind, hence, total control. We're not intrinsically the victims of so-called subconscious sabotage, primitive animal brainstem reflexes, or drives, impulses, and emotions all having a life of their own. Our bodies are purpose-built 'avatars' for emergent ℒife over which we're capable of absolute integration. Everything we think, feel, experience, and have awareness of in the physical world arises in and emanates from mind regardless our conscious or even sensorial awareness of it. This doesn't mean the physical world is an illusion but that its *existence* only has *reality* in our mind and not in and of itself, because a human person—in our case, Mina—Intentionalizes a universe into existence.

As an analogy, consider conscious awareness like a water spider prancing hither and yon across the deeper pond that is subconscious. It is separated from experiencing the deeper pond's reality by the water's surface tension, which is like mindset. Down in that pond is who you really are (fundamentally feeling, wanting, perceiving own-self and environment) generating all the currents, eddies, temperatures, and energies the water spider only dimly perceives on the surface unless the deeper environment agitates its placid footing (a person in relation to society is similar; SOL § 4:291). Conscious mind, like the water spider, is generally aware of only itself, not the depths from which it springs, because of its many segmented states of being and states of awareness upon which it focuses.

But don't think that unlocking human physiological perfection reveals all. Even if one has 100% conscious awareness of subconscious, its infinite nature means it's always beyond the scope of full awareness that conscious mind can experience. No matter how much more conscious awareness of it that one develops, there yet remains infinite unawareness of self despite omniscience of mind. One fully experiences subconscious only in the naturally segmental conscious mind. That's the awesome emergent reality of *your* mind. Love, for example, is not some magical force searing into our lives like a bolt from the blue. It's *our own (subconscious) Life force* so strongly manifesting its self-aware proto-energy reaction to an object of love's self-aware proto-energy Way of Being that it roils—perturbs—conscious awareness, and we experience its interaction.

2.2.1 Subconscious Intentionality Exerts Change on Conscious Mind

The above process is how my subconscious awareness and conscious sub-Thought (*Fig. 3.2*; SOL § 1.1.2.1:393) exerted change in my environment by Intentionalizing changes in my brain leading to pre-diagnosable early-onset dementia. It's true that when I discovered the cause of my memory issues, I was angry and rejected it out of hand. But, until that moment, my subconscious had brought my conscious mind's Thought and sub-Thought into harmony with it such that, as a wholistic person, I had a consistent attitude toward life as something to negate.

The *sub-Thought* aspect of *phyiscally instantiated* conscious mind provides the material for conscious Thought to draw upon which, recall, is thinking–feeling. Our thinking and emotional expression consciously arises here, although its emotive energy (EmℒF; CH. 4 § 1.3.1:123) arises in subconscious state of awareness and state of being. Everything that mind experiences in its subconscious (neutral) aspect reposits here in individual states of awareness and states of being like a reservoir. This is similar to the way individual action potentials—nerve impulses—aggregate into a state of being 'reservoir' from which the brain draws to form an aggregate action potential that ultimately provokes a brain–body response (SOL § 1.2.2.1:253). When a person is thinking or emoting, they draw all its Thought aspects from this aspect of conscious mind. The nature of this aspect we call sub-Thought in the context of physically instantiated albeit not ℒife mind.

Building on what people think of as self-sabotage with the example above, one's subconscious influences conscious mind to think, feel, act, and embody one's subconscious experience rather than that of conscious mind's totality of its real world environment (*Fig. 3.2*). This is so even when it contradicts conscious mind's sub-Thought and Thought. This

SUBCONSCIOUS INTENTIONALITY EXERTS ON CONSCIOUS MIND 111

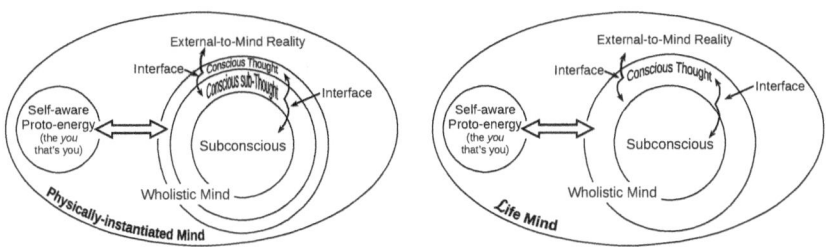

Fig. 3.2. Left, physical body: conscious sub-Thought interfaces twixt subconscious and wholistic conscious mind (sub-Thought and Thought); conscious Thought interfaces twixt wholistic mind and external-to-mind reality; right, emergent self: no sub-Thought with 𝓛ife mind.

is the reason we can't do things we tell ourselves we want to do, or do things we tell ourselves we don't want to do. In all cases, wholistic mind is achieving *reconciliation* in resolving internal inconsistency in accord with our fundamental experience of awareness, whether arising first in Thought, sub-Thought, or subconscious (*SOL* § 2.3:398).

Emergent 𝓛ife is a self-contained, self-aware proto-energy being emergently birthing 'in' Energent proto-life (*SOL* § 2.3.2.1:241). It is discrete with respect to the Energent proto-energy around it in the same way an archí—fundamental 'energy' that manifests as matter–Energy (matter)—constituting non-aware proto-energy is discrete with respect to the proto-energy around it. Your beingness, therefore, can't directly experience external-to-mind reality any more than the proto-energy contained within the archí 'shell' can. An interface is necessary. For the archí, that interface is the 'energetic' Way of Being of its 'shell' that interacts via motion with proto-energy. Similarly, we can think of subconscious–conscious mind as the 'shell' that encapsulates the ℘erson—the self-aware being having 𝓛ife—which, owing to its Intentionalized Way of Being, interfaces wholistic mind with external-to-mind existence which you experience as reality.

The sub-Thought aspect of conscious mind altogether reflects wholistically subconscious and conscious Thought's SOB–SOA. Because these states of being and states of awareness wholistically integrate, there can be no dichotomy even if there is one between these and conscious Thought's SOB–SOA. For example, let's say a person consciously experiences (thinks–feels) ABC about something while subconsciously having awareness of it as XYZ. Absent any effort on the individual's part to persuade subconscious to adopt conscious Thought's ABC thinking–feeling, subconscious exerts on conscious sub-Thought the Intentionality that naturally arises in its XYZ awareness. This has the effect of persuading the individual to think–feel in XYZ terms in sub-Thought. Thus, any thoughts, feelings, and actions not focused on conscious Thought's ABC thinking–feeling will be the xyz awareness that arose in his or her subconscious. This gives rise to our tendency to do or say things 'without thinking' to which we blurt, "I don't know why I just did [said] that," or to experience our conscience (*SOL* § 2.3:398), and so on. This happens because it's what one *really* thinks–feels when conscious Thought isn't running interference.

Section 3
Intentionality

As touched on above, Intentionality is a subconscious–emergent self function, it being the fundamental aspect of awareness of one's self-aware proto-energy self having Intentionality. Recall that your self-aware proto-energy self Intentionalizes subconscious–conscious mind into existence about three months after emergent birth as an Intentionalized Way of Being of one's self (*Fig. 3.1* on page 97). It therefore doesn't possess Intentionality as its own Way of Being any more than a universe possesses its builder's Intentional Way of Being.

However, because conscious mind is the emergent person's gateway to external-to-mind reality, Intentionality exerts external-to-mind because of it. The reason is that conscious mind's experience of external-to mind 'energies' is a two-way street with subconscious mind's awareness. Because of Intentionality, which arises 'in' proto-energy and exerts 'on' proto-energy, mind's awareness–experience of external-to-mind proto-energy means that said proto-energy is 'aware' of mind. Thusly, it responds to Intentionality.

When conscious Thought Intention is out-of-sync with subconscious Intention, Intentionality fails (*SOL* § 2.1.5.4:316). If Mina, for instance, hadn't really (subconsciously) wanted to build a universe but only (consciously) thought he did, his Intention would've failed regardless his effort. Had my subconscious awareness not been my conscious mind's encounters as a negation of physical life, it never would've Intentionalized early-onset dementia. If your body is not healthy, it's because your conscious Intention to be healthy shipwrecked on the rock of your subconscious.

Section 4
The Bell of the Mind

Let's consider exactly how it is that your subconscious Intentionally affects your physical body regardless your conscious resistance to illness, disease, chronic injury, aging effects, and the like.

4.1 The Way of 'Energy'

Recall that you are an 'energy' being. You may be tempted to think that that's because you are mind. But mind is only a *self-Intentionalized—self-actualized—aspect* of what you fundamentally are. Your mind, an Intentionality of your emergently birthed self, is like a universe which itself is a human-Intentionalized aspect of All Existence. And, like All Existence, your mind is time and space indeterminate (*Fig. 2.1:31; SOL § 2.2.1:395; SOL § 2:593*). Via your mind interface, you are exquisitely aware of every speck of 'energy' not only in your immediate surroundings but throughout our universe. Of course, farther 'energy' is more subtly encountered and experienced than nearer 'energy,' which is what we discuss in this book.

As a discrete being of 'energy,' we exist *surrounded by* 'energy.' In our physical embodiment, we exist *suffused in* 'energy.' All kinds of 'energy.' Proto-energy. Emotive energy (emotive ℒife force, or, EMℒF). Fundamental force. Applied energy E (e.g., electromagnetic). Our self-aware proto-energy self—the *you* that is you—and subconscious–conscious never *don't* encounter and experience 'energy.' Let's take, for instance, the energy of a room. You not only sense it but viscerally respond to (encountering) it and subconsciously react to (experiencing) it even before you're consciously aware of it. This is an aspect of the so-called sixth sense.

In this 'energy' milieu, think of your essential beingness like a bell that unceasingly rings a 'tone' that is your unique 'tone.' It's your emergently unique 'sound' in the universe. At the moment of your emergent birth—this is your conception in the physical embodiment context—your emergent Way of Being is wholly unique amongst humanity and the universe. No matter how many humans emergently birth across time, the 'energy' of your Way of Being is non-duplicable. The reason is that it's *emergent*. When conception triggered your emergent birth 'in' Energent proto-life, your Way of Being spontaneously—emergently—coalesced, differentiated, and self-organized. This is the very definition of emergence in the human context: a birth of ℌuman unique to All Existence. That unique ℌuman is you.

As you encounter humanity and the universe since emergent birth, you encounter the 'energy' we've mentioned above hundreds of times per second. From the instant you as a ℘erson self-Intentionalized your mind into existence, your essential self was aware of the 'energy' beyond the confines of your self-aware proto-energy beingness. You're never not aware of it. This 'energy' rings your bell the way, say, a person standing next to a church bell bangs a hammer of a particular weight, density, and material against it even as its clapper continues ringing the bell's own tone. The sound you then hear is the original sound of the bell—the 'energy' of emergent Way of Being—added to the extraneous sound of the hammer striking the bell—the 'energy' of your attributive Way of Being. The tones merge; maybe it's sharp or flat, deeper or lighter, harmonious or clashing.

If you depart from where that 'energy' is—here, we're talking about you as a physically-embodied person, not simply unembodied mind—then it rings your bell less and less until its proximity is too weak for it. However, your proto-energy self continues to ring with that added 'tone' until it dissipates, though it never dwindles to zero absent your intervention to neutralize—negate—it. Your proto-energy self always rings with your original 'tone' from before encountering that 'energy' in addition to the dissipated-but-not-zeroed-out 'tone' you encountered. This goes on every second since self-Intentionalizing your mind following emergent birth. As 'energy,' it will always be a part of the larger 'energy' matrix that is you (absent you consciously neutralizing it).

This 'energy,' which you encounter hundreds of times per second, can harmonize or clash with the 'energy' of your overall Way of Being. For example, you may encounter a person whose 'energy' rings your bell in such a way that you feel instant attraction or repulsion to some degree. This is the origin of experiencing the mystery of love and of instant revulsion (ranging from dislike to hate), respectively. Such 'energy' not only arises in people or things but also in ideas, feelings, and beliefs. Your belief that the whims of biological infection, chronic or incurable damage and illness, and the effects of aging are inevitable and unavoidable is itself an 'energy' that rang the bell of your mind from emergent birth and thereafter.

> **Side note.** The 'energy' of the universe affects you even before your self-aware proto-energy self Intentionalizes your subconscious–conscious mind at about three months following emergent birth as the interface between own-self and the universe beyond own-self (CH. 1 SELF-AWARENESS:5; *SOL* § 2:275). We'll use an applied energy E metaphor to help visualize why.
>
> Imagine that you, a new emergent birth still a fetal human without subconscious–conscious mind (*Fig. 3.1* on page 97, *right*), are an enclosed vessel of water. Sound waves from the world outside this vessel continually strike the walls of the vessel. These impart energy that interacts with the water inside the vessel—you—and accordingly set up energy waves within it. These waves have different frequency, wavelength, and amplitude from the sound waves outside the vessel that caused them. For example, a person outside the water of a swimming pool shouting at you beneath the water exemplifies this difference; you can hear sound of a sort but nothing more. Nevertheless, these waves are energy which interact with and affect the water of the vessel in a myriad of microscopic and macroscopic ways.
>
> And so it is that the 'energy' of the universe affects your self-aware proto-energy self even before you've Intentionalized your subconscious–conscious mind to directly–indirectly

experience–encounter it. However, we don't further cover this nuanced aspect in this book. Our discussion here is in the context of your subconscious–conscious mind. For more, read *SOL* CH. 26:391.

Harmonious or discordant, your subconscious *experiences* the 'energy' that your proto-energy self only *encounters*. Your proto-energy self is *aware and self-aware*, but *not experiential*. That's the province of your subconscious and is the origin of emotion. Thought (thinking–feeling) is your subconscious–conscious response to whatever you encounter. Your conscious mind parses and analyzes what your subconscious only experiences. This is why emotion seems so uncontrollable, mysterious, and visceral. It is entirely experiential, redolent—in the sense of expressive—with impression. No matter how hard you assert conscious reason, you can never remove the *experience* of your subconscious. Trying to do so only provokes a dichotomy in the mind arising in its unreconciled subconscious–conscious mindstate that eventually leads to disturbances like PTSD.

4.2 How Your Subconscious Experiences 'Energy'

For example, when your proto-energy self encounters 'energy' that clashes with the energy pattern of your proto-energy, the clash creates discordant 'energy' that bangs around your proto-energy self. You have awareness and self-awareness of 'energy,' whether it's harmonizing or discordant. There are three kinds of 'energy' of which your proto-energy self has awareness: harmonizing, discordant, and outside of self (which can be neutral). Your proto-energy self has an 'energy' reaction to any of these three kinds, and that reaction is what your subconscious experiences. That experience automatically Intentionalizes inside the mind and sometimes outside the mind as well, meaning into the world. For instance, it could be directed at the source of the 'energy' and cause harm of some kind in the case of discordant 'energy' or a draw or good feelings in the case of attraction.

If the subconscious experience is strong enough, it influences your conscious mind, meaning conscious Thought. If it's not strong enough, it stays in your subconscious and subtly influences your affect. But aspects can also percolate up to your conscious mind to influence conscious Thought thus choices hence behavior.

Your proto-energy self only experiences 'energy' outside mind via its mind interface. Without mind, your proto-energy self is insulated from the 'energy' outside mind thus outside the proto-energy self except in the aspect discussed in the SIDE NOTE on the facing page. In this case, you would simply exist within your own being having no awareness or knowledge of what's outside own-self. That's the way Mike and Molly were before they imagined the existence of another person or, later, finding and interacting with the other. They didn't know they had a mind nor that they could even use it until thinking about potential existences beyond themselves and discovering their mind Intentionally responding to Thought.

People like you and me, born after Mike and Molly thus enculturating a certain human (*vs.* Ꮈuman) Way of Being, emergently birthed into an 'energy' milieu already implanted with that previously developed Way of Being. When such a person emergently births and then intentionalizes their own mind into existence in the context of Mike and Molly's foundational (*vs.* Ꮈuman) Way of Being, *having* a mind and *knowing of* that mind lets one use it to encounter and experience All Existence beyond oneself. The 'energy' of that Way of Being ultimately formed the genesis of universal culture (Ultraculture), which affects every subsequent emergently birthed person . . . for instance, in terms of male–female sex differentiation.

Your proto-energy self cannot avoid 'energy' ringing its bell via mind. According to how subconscious experiences and reacts to that 'energy,' it resonates in your mind to cause harm or disruption or ecstasy or joy or whatever. The proto-energy self is like a bell always ringing a certain 'tone' according to the person; you can think of it, too, like an energy matrix or energy frequency. When a new 'sound' is introduced from outside via mind that, for example, roils the proto-energy self, meaning it roils the 'tone'—energy frequency—then the person experiences distress and stress and other issues in the subconscious.

If the energy is problematic in any way and it roils, or perturbs, the subconscious because it roils the proto-energy self (being in conflict with the 'energy' of the person's emergent Way of Being), then the person experiences inner conflict. If this new 'energy' overwhelms the 'energy' of emergent Way of Being, you settle down to a new Way of Being that's of your original 'energy' plus this new 'energy,' which is a new 'frequency,' or 'tone,' for you. Eventually, it percolates up through the subconscious to conscious mind to affect Thought thus behavior. If it doesn't overwhelm emergent Way of Being, then it becomes a subtle source of inner conflict that's unresolvable until you consciously take control to neutralize—negate—that 'energy' in your subconscious, thus your proto-energy self. The subconscious doesn't initiate this, only conscious mind does.

As you emergently birth and grow up experiencing the 'energy' of the universe and all humanity within it, you encounter all kinds of problematic 'energies.' (We point out that problematic 'energies' are a natural part of

Life because human beings are absolutely autonomous.) To the degree your subconscious experiences these 'energies' rather than rejecting or moderating them then, over time, it overwhelms emergent Way of Being and you become a person of a different Way of Being. Rejecting or moderating such 'energies' means your own subconscious rings your subconscious bell to effectively cancel the 'vibration,' 'wave,' and so on, the way out-of-phase sound waves negate each other. This is conscious mind having retrained your Intentional proto-energy self therefore subconscious to operate in accord with emergent Way of Being, thus acting as a shield.

For example, the 'energy' of emergent—at emergent birth—Way of Being is that your physical body does not age nor is affected by the 'energy' of biology (recall that everything is 'energy,' even ideas, beliefs, and attitudes). However, being born into the physical world having no awareness of your physicospirit existence, you come to accept all the 'energy' of the world. These 'energies' overwhelm the 'energy' of emergent Way of Being with the 'energy' of a new Way of Being in which you're a biological entity and totally susceptible to the vagaries of biology in the same way as nonhuman entities. These become subconscious 'beliefs,' your mindset. They are constantly Intentionalized by your emergent self via subconscious, which is an Intentional—self-actualizing—machine.

Because you mind–brain and mind–body integrate your body, your Intentional self ever Intentionalizes into body all the 'energy' it experiences to greater or lesser degrees since body *is* emergent self. There is no distinction between itself and body. They are one and the same. This is how your body comes to manifest aging, chronic injury, susceptibility to illness and disease, and the like. While your subconscious can work like a shield to avoid 'energy' pinging your subconscious bell, your best defense is to have no subconscious 'belief' that accepts external 'energy' harming your body. In practical terms, this means your subconscious does not Intentionally negate your body's emergent Way of Being. Recall that we generally typeset traditional subconscious belief as 'belief,' which means a reality that your mind accepts as *an 'energy' awareness that may or may not Intentionalize.*

Section 5
Conclusion to Chapter 3

To sum up, mind is subconscious–conscious and is different from psyche (consciousness). As wild as it seems, *you*—your emergent self-aware proto-energy self—spontaneously self-Intentionalized your mind at about three months following emergent birth (conception). Your emergent self via subconscious is who you are. It's your who-ness and constitutes around 99.996% of wholistic mind. You are not conscious mind, the environment of your external-to-mind experience, inner voice, and thinking–feeling. You are subconscious (an aspect of self-aware proto-energy), the environment of your awareness, ideas, drive, ambition, and Way of Being. Subconscious is emergently self-aware and not the same thing as conscious mind. It's fundamental of Ꜧuman. A person is neither mind nor cognition but awareness. Subconscious 'belief' is a reality—an 'energy' awareness—that you accept as real that typically Intentionalizes damage into your body.

Your subconscious is like a bell, which 'energy' pings. It then vibrates a 'tone' inclusive of the existing 'tone' throughout your mind thus your body. The bell which 'energy' pings is the self-aware proto-energy self, the Intentional origin of mind which encounters and objectively experiences 'energy.' It's always Intentionalizing; it's never not Intentionalizing. The instant your subconscious experiences 'energy,' that 'energy' enters an Intentional state in your emergent self. Accordingly, your emergent self via subconscious ceaselessly Intentionalizes its encounters with 'energy' as a literal reality into your life, your body, and sometimes your environs. This Intentional 'energy' continually exerting on your body provokes and maintains the malfunctions that people think of as health issues, aging, and death.

In the next chapter, we describe how your Intentional self creates the physical reality that your body encounters as a malfunction.

How the Body Malfunctions

Your body is not animal. It is human. This means your body was empowered to integrate a human mind. Absent that integrated mind, which is you, the person, your body indeed is as animal as a monkey. We call such a physical body *proto-human*, a 𝕃iving entity: the anatomically and pre-anatomically correct human body prior to ℒife integrating it on Earth about 50,000 years ago (sol § 2.1.2:543) not to mention your own two-cell zygote. Once integrated, your body is 𝔥uman. The reason is that, when it comes to anything human, we aren't talking interaction, interrelationship, sharing, inhabiting, or the like, but *integration*.

Our mind—our self-aware proto-energy self—doesn't *inhabit* our physical body but *integrates*. Integration is *amalgamation* in the sense of alloy as an admixture where entities retain their individual properties. Think of two objects coming closer together, touching, then amalgamating into a single form yet remaining discrete (sol § 1.2.2.3:256). This transforms the body from 𝕃iving to ℒife.

Accordingly and despite your physical body being a physical entity in and of itself, it is an extension of your mind. It *is* your mind. It therefore reflects your mind in every way. Your emergent self via subconscious constitutes about 99.996% of wholistic mind (forget the conventional visible–invisible iceberg metaphor). What happens in the self happens in the body; there's no what-happens-in-Vegas-stays-in-Vegas here.

Philosophy with a capital-P in some of its spiritual incarnations sometimes says the human person is only a spiritual being and therefore the body isn't real. Or that the sensation of living matter is an illusion, that it's all in your mind. But there is sensation in matter because your body is also a Living entity just like an animal (even a plant, which evidences sensation, too; *Secret Life,* Tompkins).

To comprehend this in the human context, we need recognize that mind integrates brain and emergent self integrates body. Therefore, until you have full awareness that your body *is* your emergent proto-energy incorporating emergent Way of Being then you inevitably, meaning subconsciously, choose to Intentionally experience the 'energy' of damage to your body inclusive of physical damage like broken bones as attributive Way of Being. This attributive subconscious 'energy' Intentionalizes into your body, the reality of which physically manifests.

With full awareness of physicospirit existence—you as physically alive plus your spirit embodied self—your emergent self does not Intentionalize the 'energy' of damage into your body. It thereby does not manifest in your body. Making the sensations of your body an experience of reality makes it attributive Way of Being because your emergent self is Intentionalizing into your body what you accept as reality in your mind. This includes pain.

As your awareness grows, you clear this attributive Way of Being from your body as easily as you change your thoughts until your body *is* the 'energy' of your emergent proto-energy incorporating emergent Way of Being. This is your awareness of the supremacy of mind over matter, which is true because you are an Intentional being, not an animal. This awareness governs your ability to Intentionalize good health and wellbeing. (Keep in mind that wishful thinking is not Intentional Thought but only an intention or desire; it needs Intentional energy to become Intentionality.) With such awareness, you no longer need feel alarmed, as damage no longer harms you. This happens because your physical body (integrating *L*ife, which emergently birthed as emergent proto-energy 'in' Energent proto-life) is healthy and complete *as* emergent Way of Being.

We're used to thinking that our conscious mind is our conscious*ness*, who we are. This is an inaccurate observation born of our inability to perceive our physicospirit reality. All of our thinking–feeling (Thought) originates as a wholistic state of being (SOB) and state of awareness (SOA) in the subconscious that Intentionalizes literally infinite states of being and states of awareness to the conscious mind where we parse them into what people think of as everyday thought and emotion.

Recall that SOA refers to the awareness one has in totality with respect to what's of interest and SOB is one's experience of the referent SOA (CH. 2 § 4.1.1:70). Also, that subconscious awareness is not only too fast for our brain to operate on, its mode of awareness is incompatible with brain's cognitive function. Thus, it requires transliteration from one environment to the other. This is mind–brain integration.

We noted in CH. 2 § 4.3.1 on page 76 that The Corruption interfered with mindset and, ultimately, mind–brain integration. This caused a mental blindness as well as a structural limitation in the brain restricting how much mind integrates it at any given moment, which prevents awareness (*SOL* § 1.2.2.5:261). Its effect physically cut off humanity from the fullness of *Life*; we're unable to experience most of our own emergent *Life* states of being and states of awareness.

For example, we experience some of the primitive reflexes, drives, impulses, and awareness redolent with impression of our proto-human past because of The Corruption. Still, an individual capably has full awareness thus total control of his or her mind therefore body. Our subconscious doesn't sabotage us. It's literally who we are. Conscious mind is only an expression of subconscious. Your body was empowered to integrate emergent *Life*; you are capable of absolute integration. Whatever you think, feel, experience, and have awareness of in your physical embodiment arises in and emanates from your emergent *Life* mind regardless your conscious awareness of or sensorial experience with it.

Still, we certainly do experience all the vagaries of biological existence—malfunctions—that animals do. This seemingly makes the case that humans are nothing more than biological entities. That is inaccurate, however. Toward explaining why, we describe in this chapter the three categories of malfunction: damage/injury, aging, and death.

Section 1
Damage/Injury

1.1 Damage

Damage is any physical impact or physical change that creates a disruption in the body. This could be a vehicle crash, a pressure wave, a fall (well, the landing), a separation twixt things normally joined (cut, tear, break), cellular/DNA metamorphosis, or a destructive biological, chemical, or radiological exposure.

1.2 Injury

Injury is any damage caused by Intentionalized 'energy' from your or another's subconscious. This is either subconsciously in the traditional sense as consciously unintended, or as motivated by conscious Thought such as a curse—merely a particular kind of Intentionality—or any conscious Intention to inflict harm. Injury as *'energy' trauma* is the effect of damage to one's body or injury to one's mind via 'energy' rather than damage as described above. Damage in this context is Intentionalized 'energy' gaslighting your subconscious to Intentionalize it as 'energy' of damage—attributive Way of Being—in the targeted part of your body, which affects the energy pattern thereof and leads to malfunctions—damage—that degrade the function of the affected area.

Injury in this context is the effect of 'energy' ringing the bell of the mind such that mind changes its Way of Being to embody the 'energy' trauma as its new Way of Being. For instance, you're feeling all young and invincible. Then you are 'energy' attacked by the 'energy' of beliefs, thoughts, ideas, culture, or even a person. The effect of that 'energy' on your Way of Being translates to a subconsciously Intentionalized malfunction of your body that leads you to a subconscious 'belief'—attributive Way of Being—that you aren't invincible. That you'll age. Have chronic injury in the form of incurable disease or damage, and so forth. An example of this is luridly describing seasick symptoms to another who's feeling fine but consequently internalizes then experiences the symptoms.

Such 'energy' assaults, not necessarily Intentionalized by another person but more often absorbed from humanity's Ultraculture on Earth, happen from your emergent birth but more profoundly from Day One of your self-aware proto-energy self Intentionalizing your subconscious–conscious mind into existence at about three months after emergent birth (CH. 3 § 1:95). Prior to your mind interacting with existence outside of mind, you were affected by albeit unaware of such 'energies.' *Ultraculture* is the universal culture of our universe. It's the state of being and Way of Being of all humans and nonhumans, and ever so subtly spans all minds.

1.3 Why Disease

Disease for animals is beyond their individual and collective control whereas for humans it is not. This means it's necessarily not an immutable biological inevitability. For you, as human, the effects of disease arise exclusively in subconscious–conscious 'belief'—the 'energy' of attributive Way of

Being—that becomes mindset, which the Intentional power of subconscious manifests into physical reality.

Recall that Intentionality is your exerted subconscious experience which interacts with Energent proto-energy permeating our universe. This Intentionalized 'energy' has an energy pattern that rings the bell of your mind. Its Intentionalized energy pattern changes the energy pattern—the 'tone'—of your body. This new energy pattern then becomes your body's new energy pattern—its amalgamated 'tone'—thus determining how your body functions or malfunctions. Intentionality affects your body as a whole or specific parts or aspects of it.

Intentionalized emotive energy (emotive ℒife force; EmℒF; *below*) is one aspect of Intentionality. Unlike Intentionalized Thought, this 'energy' gets localized to parts of your body where it constantly changes the energy pattern of that part. Your emergent self then reacts Intentionally to that 'energy' as described above. At the same time, the energy pattern of emergent Way of Being also exerts in that part of your body. When it exerts more strongly than localized Intentional EmℒF plus the 'energy' of attributive Way of Being, this is what people call natural healing. When it doesn't, it means these two energy patterns have exerted more strongly than the energy pattern of emergent Way of Being in that part of your body. It consequently manifests these energy patterns instead.

The above interferes with the proper working of that aspect of your body and leads to a malfunction, which is what people call short-term or chronic damage and illness. This is why you have disease and chronic health problems. The effect of aging is nothing more than chronic damage.

1.3.1 Emotive Expression: Emotive ℒife Force

Let's consider Emotive ℒife force. Ever wonder why one can enter a space and 'feel the atmosphere'? Why some folks are empaths? Why children (even animals) respond not to words but the emotive content of voice, expression, or affect? Why panic or (un)happiness is contagious? Why plants experience felt-hate or thoughts of violence from another room? The reason is ℒife and ℒiving force. The same force that manifests Intentionality and proto-love also manifests feeling 'in' the Energent proto-energy suffusing ℒife, the person. So-called emotional, or emotive, energy is simply one's self-aware proto-energy beingness Intentionalized by emotion, which is Thought thus 'energy.' In the context of humans, *The Story of ℒife* calls this 'energy' *emotive ℒife force* (EmℒF; SOL § 3.3.3.1.1:289).

Normatively felt emotion—EmℒF—encases us 'energetically' in the same way people imagine that auras, chakras, and bioenergy do. It's a sort of 'energy' bubble normally extending about a foot from our form. It's functionally a neutral state. This means it doesn't 'energize'—Intentionalize—proto-energy; that's just how it is. Howsoever intensely we feel so-called positive emotion, and the happiest we can ever imagine feeling, that's just normative. Yet, the happiest you've ever felt never matches your worst. This is because happiness, generally considered an emotively positive state of being conveying a sense of general wellbeing, is part of our base disposition, i.e., emergent Way of Being. Therefore, EmℒF exudes normatively—it doesn't 'energize,' i.e., Intentionalize, proto-energy—from our physical body into the ambient proto-energy environment no more than about a foot on average. This so-called positive emotive state is called happiness, but it's merely ℒife's natural state. Absent negative emotion, it's how we are. This means that humanity has never even approached its emotive norm.

On the other hand, although negative emotion is a natural aspect of ℒife, it's not our normative disposition. It deviates from ℒife's Way of Being the way a rainsquall—an inevitable, periodic necessity—deviates from the environment's base disposition of calm, neutral weather. Thus, people feel negative emotion far more intensely than positive emotion. Because it isn't normative—neutral—like positive emotion, negative emotion always Intentionalizes. The greater the intensity of our negative feeling, the greater the Intentionality experienced by Energent proto-energy outside our body and, therefore, the greater the swath of proto-energy a person's negative EmℒF 'energizes.'

Negative emotion includes more than fear, worry, hurt, heartbreak, or depression as individual feelings. Each feeling individually instantiates infinite combinations with others of varying intensities. These mix and match into an emotional gruel that's a generalized unhappy state of being. The outcome is an emotive state of greater intensity than our normative disposition because we feel this deviant state of being so painfully. This means that negative EmℒF is better conceptualized as *harmful* EmℒF in that harm doesn't arise in neutral EmℒF. This is what traditionally negative feeling is. We stick with the strong, traditional connotation for clarity but keep in mind that, to the degree our subconscious does not neutralize negative EmℒF, it is harmful EmℒF and, therefore, harmful 'energy.'

In consequence of the foregoing, negative EmℒF 'energizes' the ambient proto-energy of the Energent around a person far more intensely. It reaches farther out from their presence where other people encounter it. If they're sufficiently sensitive, like an empath, they experience it. This is why empaths experience only negative feeling. No empath feels inexplicably happy or joyful; soft science research that indicates empaths feel happiness when someone else is happy is, in truth, merely the empath's greater sensitivity to *neutral* EM⌁F than the average (non-empathic) person in the context where the absence of negative EM⌁F manifests a stark difference for the empath.

Rather, empaths struggle—particularly those who are unaware they're empaths—with negative feelings like depression, angst, anger, fear, sorrow, and so on which they mistake as their own. Such feeling can be so intense it drives some to suicide, drugs, or aberrant behavior among other effects. Unaware empaths don't realize 'their' feelings originate with others who are in physical or spirit proximity, where proximity defines an area of sensitivity; it could be an entire city or the whole planet including the 'reflective' environment. See *The Story of Life* § 3.3.3.1.1.1:290 for a bit more discussion on empaths.

1.4 Why Aging?

The effects of aging—a change in function, which is injury as above—is the normal Way of Being for most animals but not for humans.

> **Side Note.** Where humanity has full mind–brain integration (MBI), it collectively or individually Intentionalizes certain animals' lifespans, particularly those to which humans tend to bond. Even with humanity's current ∼40% average MBI (up from ∼30% since the Big Healing October 13, 2017; *TBH*, *SOL* CH. 4; *SOL* § 4:377), individuals subconsciously Intentionalize the lifespans of animals with which they bond to be somewhat longer or shorter than a species' norm the same way they Intentionalize their own life spans (outside physical damage but in keeping with subconscious 'belief;' CH. 4 § 1.1:121). People can bond with any nonhuman creature, but there are *companion animals*—dogs, cats, horses, etc. (*SOL* CH. 39:601)—that Mina created for that purpose. These lack a naturally normative life span like, say, cockroaches or amoeba.

For us, the effect of aging is both 'belief' and mindset. Recall that *'belief'* is an Intentionalized reality of subconscious 'energy,' which we typeset in single quotes to distinguish it from the traditional concept of subconscious belief. A *mindset* is a collection of such 'beliefs.' You can have 'beliefs' that are not part of your mindset and a mindset that does not embody all of your 'beliefs.' All physical persons on Earth have a 'belief' in the reality and inevitability of the effects of aging. But not every person's mindset embodies that 'belief.' These are the people who more slowly show the effects of aging and tend to live longer or healthier despite traditionally harmful lifestyles like cigarette smoking (usually chalked up to "he [she] has good genes").

The effects of aging exists for humans because of 'belief' and mindset. Even if you personally don't have a subconscious–conscious 'belief' that the effects of aging are inevitable and immutable, humanity's collective 'belief' and mindset suffuse your subconscious with Intentional effect as with any 'energy' that rings the bell of your mind. It therefore Intentionalizes that reality into your body regardless because, remember, body *is* emergent self.

Thus, aging is the Intentionalized effect of injury to your body that results in damage. But you can reverse it by removing that 'belief' and mindset as well as by letting go, in your subconscious, of humanity's collective 'belief' and mindset with respect to aging (CH. 8 § 2:172). From there, your body only needs manifest *Life* force—emergent proto-energy incorporating emergent Way of Being—which is to say, healing.

1.5 Why Death?

Your physical body—not *you*, the self-aware proto-energy person—dies because the collective mindset of physical humanity has that 'belief.' It encompasses the collective human mindset which then embodies in your life experience. Death happens regardless of age and any damage inclusive of injury because your subconscious has the 'belief' that it's time (or you subconsciously desire) for your body to die.

For example, it's not the cancer or the bullet that shuts down your organs and leads to death but your subconscious. If your subconscious isn't ready for your body to die then it mitigates the cancer or bullet damage to some degree within the bounds of its 'belief' and mindset regarding these so that your organs continue functioning and you gain some more time. If something happens during this period to alter your 'belief,' then you can have what people think of as a miraculous remission of cancer or survive a seemingly fatal bullet wound. Or, conversely, you might experience unexpectedly sudden death. If your subconscious doesn't alter its 'belief' then, regardless sufficient medical intervention, it continues to metastasize through your body and doctors say, "Well, it's a particularly aggressive cancer," or "It unexpectedly turned out to be a fatal wound." Oncologists Ernest and Isadora Rosenbaum put it this way in "The Will to Live" (2024):

> Sometimes the biology of a cancer will dictate the course of events regardless of the patient's attitude and fighting spirit . . . [and] are often beyond our control . . . Many physicians have seen how two patients of similar ages and with the same diagnosis, degree of illness, and

treatment program experience vastly different results. One of the few apparent differences is that one patient is pessimistic and the other optimistic . . . [Since] the writings of Plato and Galen . . . there is a direct correlation between the mind, the body, and one's health. "The cure of many diseases is unknown to physicians," Plato concluded, "because they are ignorant of the whole. For the part can never be well unless the whole is well" . . . [T]he psychological and the physical elements of a body are not separate, isolated, and unrelated, but are vitally linked elements of a total system . . . [H]owever diverse they are in ethnic or cultural background, age, educational level, or type of illness, they have all gone through a similar process of psychological recovery. They all consciously made a "decision to live" . . . Their "will to live" means that they really want to live, whether or not they're afraid to die. (par. 2–10)

The Rosenbaums are talking about Intentionality, here. But on the other side of things, one can be mildly damaged in some way—say, shot in the foot—yet still die owing to subconscious 'belief' that the damage is or should or desired to be fatal. Something fatal accordingly manifests, say, septicemia, and the body manifests death. Or, one subconsciously (or via their conscious spirit self) takes the opportunity to let go physical life for a better time in the Great Beyond. This is the cause of so-called death by heartbreak or losing the will to live.

Medicine considers you nothing more than animal—Living—with some kind of mysterious thought process arising in a sophisticated brain that might affect your body's health. But the "will to live" is a manifestation of conscious Thought reconciling subconscious 'belief,' thus altering Intentionality. The Intentional power of mind does the rest. Healing isn't magic. It's your own emergent self Intentionalizing your body's damage and, ultimately, its death. The *effects* of the 'energy' that Intentionally manifest in your body is what, for example, people call cancer. But you can change that. Because you are ℒife.

What Is a Malfunction

Anything that interferes with what people consider perfect physical health and wellbeing is a *malfunction*. The reason is that perfect health is your body's emergent—original—Way of Being. Recall from CH. 3 § 2.1.2.1 on page 103 that it's not biology, evolution, magic, or a deity that's the true source of your body's manifestation in the physical and spirit environments. It's your Intentional self. Your body is literally a manifestation of your emergent self in the physical context of biological matter despite it having a certain independent existence apart from mind. That is to say, procreation is a biological process of (𝕃iving) matter until the very moment your emergent birth integrates *you*, the self-aware proto-energy ℘erson, with the matter–Energy of your body as it completes second mitosis (from two cells to four).

> **Side Note.** Intentionality certainly does affect (indirectly) spirit and (directly) physical procreation even prior to fertilization (*see* SOL § 1.3.3:474).

The above isn't any different, really, than your spirit body as a manifestation of your mind in the spirit context of supramatter which, unlike physical matter, exists directly in response to mind. Your spirit body manifests from the very moment of emergent birth. It's a direct expression of your Way of Being incorporating emergent ℌuman Way of Being. Only after about three months, when your self-aware proto-energy self Intentionalizes—self-actualizes—mind as a spontaneous emergent, does subconscious–conscious exert Intentional influence on your spirit body's manifestation in concert with all the Intentional energies brought to bear by your parents and sometimes others (SIDE NOTE on the previous page).

Recall, too, that subconscious 'belief' is an Intentionalized reality of emergent self 'energy,' not the sort of beliefs you have with your conscious mind. Since your physical body reflects your mind and manifests what your subconscious 'believes'—accepts as real—about your body, then when your subconscious 'belief' embodies the 'energy' of emergent Way of Being so, too, does your body.

This book calls anything less than perfect physical health and wellbeing a *malfunction*. The reason is that, through subconscious 'belief' and mindset which don't express the 'energy' of emergent Way of Being and therefore negate it, *you are imposing damage on your body*. This is *attributive* Way of Being not your body's *emergent* Way of Being, its emergent function. Thus, your body necessarily functions in accord with attributive Way of Being because, being Intentionality, it negates the 'energy' of emergent Way of Being's effect, which is not Intentionality. Such damage is a malfunction since your body is empowered to integrate mind for which damage is emergently alien. Lacking awareness of physicospirit reality, humanity has heretofore believed its physical existence was only ever malfunction rooted in sin (spiritualism) or biology (materialism–physicalism).

Unlike nonhumans, you integrate your body as a mind–brain and mind–body amalgamation. Integration is Intentional. It's your emergent self exerting ℒife force 'energy' in tandem with your body's 𝕃iving 'energy.' *Emergent self* means your fundamental, self-aware proto-energy self plus mind. ℒife force integrates and enlivens body from 𝕃iving entity to ℒife being. Mind integrates brain and establishes physically instantiated mind. Philosophy with a capital-P imagines brain as mind, but tangible brain is only intangible mind's transliterator in the physical world.

Altogether, mind–brain integration and ℒife force establish a person as physicospirit embodiment. It is in your ℒife force mind–body integration that subconscious 'belief' and mindset Intentionalize—in this case, impose—their energy patterns into your body. When subconscious 'belief' and mindset embody emergent Way of Being then your body's energy pattern necessarily manifests only perfect health. Otherwise, your body malfunctions to greater or lesser degrees according to subconsciously Intentionalized attributive Way of Being.

The matter of your body constitutes of 'energy,' hence it is matter–Energy not simply matter. Intentional subconscious–conscious means your body responds to the energy pattern set up within it from any Intentional source. There are three sources by which your body malfunctions: the 'energy' of subconscious–conscious (emergent self), the 'energy' of another person's subconscious–conscious, and the 'energy' of human Ultraculture. An important caveat here is that, regardless the origin of Intentional energy, only your subconscious–conscious mind Intentionalizes it into your body. Let's consider each one in turn.

Section 1
Intentionality From Own-self Mind

We describe *malfunction* in Chapter 4 and define it above. In this section here, we describe how you self-Intentionalize how your physical body experiences physical life.

It's not the case that your physical body is born as either a result or a victim of evolution, genetics, environment, or metabolism. This is the reality of nonhumans, not humans. Your reality is that the health of your body is altogether a result of your or others' Intentionalized 'energy' or else the 'energy' of Ultraculture. Your body conceived in accord with emergent Way of Being, which is the Way of Being of Ꜧuman. Accordingly, your physical body's Way of Being is the Way of Being of Ꜧuman. This Way of Being reflects Energent proto-life from which you emergently birthed. This means your body's Way of Being, whether emergent function or attributive malfunction, is a direct expression of subconscious 'belief' since the 'energy' of body *is* the 'energy' of emergent self.

One aspect of Energent proto-life in our universe is that it's eternal—time indeterminate—in the same way that Energent–prime proto-energy of All Existence is eternal. Therefore your physical body, which is an aspect of the same Way of Being, is also eternal. It's eternal because your self-aware proto-energy, the 'energy' that is you, is eternal. Your physical body manifests into a state of aliveness (𝕃iving) in the fertilization process just before emergent birth, after which it *is* 𝓛ife as an extension of your self-aware proto-energy self. That's your body's emergent Way of Being. But it doesn't have to be eternal if you don't want it to be since you are an absolutely autonomous being.

With full mind–brain and mind–body integration, you control your body entirely. Every aspect of biology, genetics, internal environment, all of it. Even if a bullet hits your body, you control how your body experiences that. The control you have over your body is absolute. It's determined by subconscious 'belief' and mindset which establish the 'energy' of your body right down to its DNA roots. It might seem you have no control over your body because you may believe your conscious mind controls you and that your subconscious is only the quiet swamp of your conscious waters.

For example, some American Indians believed that ghost shirts would protect them from the US Army's bullets. Unfortunateley, the Battle of Wounded Knee in 1890 proved they wouldn't. That's not because they were wrong per se. It's because conscious belief did not match subconscious 'belief' and mindset. As subconscious is 99.996% of mind, then subconscious 'belief' manifests in the body over and above conscious belief unless or until it rises to Intentionality and your emergent self Intentionally responds.

Because your body's emergent Way of Being is eternal, it's not affected by the biological reality that governs nonhumans. Your physical body has perfect health from the get-go. It can never be affected by anything that contradicts the 'energy' of emergent Way of Being except your own Intentionalized subconscious 'belief' that disease, virus, bacterial infection, chronic injury, aging until your body dies, or birth defects controls your body.

> **Side Note.** Birth defects are a manifestation of Intentional 'energy' present in the sperm or egg from damage or injury as described in CH. 4 § 1:121. Too, harmful Intentionality in the womb from the mother or another person's subconscious–conscious manifests injury that people classify as a birth defect. An otherwise healthy fetus—one not subjected to any individual's harmful Intentional 'energy'—develops a birth defect from the collective human mindset's Intentional response to particular energy patterns arising in the vagaries of biology, which themselves initially arose in the collective human mindset (Ultraculture).
>
> For example, Down's Syndrome first arose in the conscious Intention of a single spirit individual around 25,000 years ago as an attack on a specific person in the womb. As it manifested, other spirit persons took note and later Intentionalized its energy pattern for their own purposes. Over time, the presence of this malady entered the collective human mindset. As a collective belief strengthened that a baby could be born with it, the collective human mindset's Intentional response to that energy pattern also strengthened until it exerted sufficient Intentional energy (CH. 6) as the focal point of the energy pattern that people identify as Down's Syndrome to manifest the problem.
>
> Over the course of 25,000 years, its energy pattern increasingly randomly manifested as the vagaries of biology, which vagaries even exist because of the effects of The Corruption on human behavior thus humanity's collective, Intentional mindset.

A malfunction happens in the discrepancy between emergent Way of Being of eternal, perfect health and your attributive Way of Being built up from the collective human mindset and your own subconscious 'belief' and mindset. Such 'belief' generally is that you're basically a smart animal subject to all biological processes like any other animal. That you can be harmed and killed by disease, illness, injury, aging, and so on. That your body must inevitably grow old into decrepitude until your organs cease to function and you die.

In this case, your attributive mindset is stronger than emergent Way of Being because your emergent self is an Intentional machine ever Intentionalizing Thought (not the everyday, ordinary thoughts of conscious mind). It constantly, unceasingly Intentionalizes subconscious 'belief' into your body, the 'energy' of which *is* emergent self regardless its own emergent Way of Being. This is how physical harm manifests in your body seemingly out of the blue without any discernible cause—for example, a sudden onset of nausea, cramps, heart issues, pain in the brain (headaches, dizziness, unconsciousness), and many more.

A person changing subconscious 'belief' to be more in accord with the 'energy' of emergent Way of Being allows the latter to successfully manifest in their body. This is the origin of the body's self-healing ability, which is a function of Living before integrating ℒife and afterward an aspect of ℒife; nonhumans have *original* Way of Being whereas humans have *emergent* Way of Being. It's also the origin of spontaneous healing, miraculous healing in the hospital, on the deathbed, in the operating room (not a near death experience, that's a different thing; SOL § 4.1.3.1:423), to survive seemingly fatal injury, and so forth. Where a person subconsciously 'believes' some particular damage is chronic, incurable, or fatal then, regardless conscious belief or desire, that damage is what your body manifests even if it's not, intrinsically in and of itself, any of those.

Section 2
Intentionality From Other-self Mind

We live in a world peopled with others. Each one is a self-aware proto-energy being of Intentional mind like you. Just as people consciously and physically harm others, they also do it subconsciously. This arises in their physicospirit embodiment where every physically alive person is simultaneously spirit embodied. In this section, we describe how another person's emergent self Intentionalizes to varying degrees how your physical body experiences physical life.

In this case, another person Intentionalizes Thought to which the proto-energy suffusing our universe as well as your physical body responds. However, it only manifests in your body as the *other* person's Intentional Thought—as some kind of harm, say—when *your* subconscious 'belief' and mindset are conducive to it having an effect. Put differently, Intentional 'energy' of damage only damages your body when your subconscious 'belief' accepts it as real and accordingly goes along with it, Intentionally making it your body's reality. However, if your subconscious 'belief' and mindset more or less embody emergent Way of Being then Intentionalized harm less or more affects your body because your subconscious rejects the attributive Way of Being of damage. If your subconscious fully embodies emergent Way of Being then Intentionalized harm from any source has no effect on your body. Zip. Nada. This is the most effective way to shield yourself from another's Intentionalized harm.

Intentional Thought not only inflicts harm but healing, too. This is how legitimate healers (e.g., Mary Baker Eddy, d. 1910) achieve healing. As with Intentionalized harm, the effect of Intentionalized healing also depends on subconscious 'belief' and mindset. If a person exerts Intentional healing on your body, for instance, it physically alters the energy pattern of your body which effects measurable healing so long as you gave permission, meaning that you want it. But if your subconscious 'belief' and mindset resists or rejects it, then healing may only be partial and temporary because your Intentional emergent self reverses—negates—the healing. This is the reason that healing requires permission; besides respecting absolute autonomy, you can't heal people who don't want it.

A healer can convey healing even when your subconscious has no 'belief' in it or actively resists it. The reason is that the healer's Intentionalized ℒife force incorporating emergent Way of Being negates your attributive Way of Being (subconscious 'belief') that subconsciously resists—acts to negate—healing. In other words, the healing Intentionality is stronger than your attributive Way of Being. It effectively modifies it such that your attributive Way of Being temporarily *is* the healing Intentionality. However, such healing is still only partial or temporary because, after a healer exerts Intentional healing into your body, your subconscious (if not your conscious) attributive Way of Being—disbelief in it or resistance to it—continually works against it. Negating it. Over time, this will undo it. Nevertheless, the more you experience physical healing, the less insistent your subconscious 'belief' resists it. You can speed your healing by Intentionally accepting its reality.

2.1 Ultraculture

Ultraculture refers to the collective consciousness—an ever-present Intentionalized 'energy' that is humanity's collective subconscious 'mind energy'—that prevails throughout our universe, thus Earth. In our universe, Ultraculture is its own unique instantiation of All Existence Ultimaculture that subtly encapsulates megaversal humanity whether embodied or unembodied. Until the Big Healing on October 13, 2017, Ultraculture was altogether negative—harmful—because of The Corruption and the Accountableism that so-called archangel Michael's Lie reinforced. Its 'energy'—emotive *Life* force interacting with proto-energy—plus those inimical to Mina's healing efforts constantly fomented unforeseen and undesirable change in the physical environment leading to creatures and biology dangerous to humans.

Mina found such constantly replenished 'energy' difficult to keep up with and eradicate across the millions of human-populated planets (SOL § 2.1.5.5.2.2:323) as well as in the supranatural environment of our universe since its origin is in the individual and collective human mind. You see, the omnipotence of a universe builder doesn't mean he or she can work (near-) instantaneous physical change nor compel free, autonomous persons to their will. Earth's sacred texts abundantly demonstrate this truth in their descriptions of humanity's omnipresent sin and rebellion to its gods. The power of a universe builder in the human context is relative, not absolute (SOL § 1:335).

Since culture is mind, it instantiates *as* mind. As states of being (SOB) and Way of Being, brainstate instantiates from singular nerve impulses—action potentials (AP)—to clades, superclades, megaclades, and ultraclades, building states of being from AP-SOB to ultraclade-SOB (SOL § 1.2.2:253). Similarly, culture instantiates from individuals as cultural vectors (CV) to CV culture, supercultures, megacultures, and ultraculture, building states of being from CV-SOB to ultraculture-SOB (SOL *Fig.* 124:292). This means culture begins in the person as states of being and Way of Being. It then instantiates amongst enmeshed persons such as two friends, family, school, job, ethnicity, community, nation, or planet until reaching its largest possible instantiation in our universe: Ultraculture. This is the universal culture of our universe, the states of being and Way of Being of all humans and nonhumans therein. Ultraculture spans all minds.

So-called human nature is nothing more than core culture amongst enmeshed—entangled—persons and is habitual, not genetic. We inherit it in the sense that such core habituations pass to children unconsciously through our states of being and Way of Beingness because individual core culture *is* states of being and Way of Being, which is 100% *of* mind. Still, one mustn't divorce what's called human nature from the emergent *Life* person. Instead, we need recognize it *as* emergent Way of Being plus attributive Way of Being (which is amenable). Our physical manifestation of ℒife is, to us, quite vague. As we lack awareness of our physicospirit reality, talking about 'human nature' is as ineffectual as speculating on the taste of moon cheese. Since only about 0.004% of mind is consciously aware (SOL § 1.2.2.1:253), it's plain that our nonconscious—sub-Thought and subconscious in the physical body context (*Fig. 3.2* on page 111)—infinite self mainly affects states of being and Way of Being.

See *The Story of ℒife* § 4:291 for a full discussion on culture generally and Ultraculture specifically. With Chapters 1–5 as a useful foundation, we now turn to Intentionality.

Intentionality

Intentionality is mind's exertion of Thought (CH. 2 § 1.3:32) into the universe such that it *embodies*, meaning it has existence in time and space. Looking back to Mike and Molly, they came to understand that whatever they thought in a certain way actually came about one way or another in their external-to-own-self environment. For example, as soon as Molly imagined there could be another self like own-self, her mind activated in a way she'd never experienced, deploying senses and 'energy' she didn't know she had until Mike experienced them. She experienced Mike in the same way.

Essentially, her exertion of mind provoked a proto-energy response 'in' Energent–prime that Mike experienced *as* awareness. He responded similarly, which Molly experienced *as* awareness. Their awareness of Intentionalized 'energy' introduced them. They experimented with this built-in feature quite a bit as they rooted down to the cellars of their minds for every functionality they could uncover (SOL § 2.1.2:308).

With time, Molly got to wondering if she could *cause to exist* something herself rather than hoping to find existents already 'outside' of her.

> **Side Note.** Molly appears to be the dynamic one in this duo. This isn't a reflection of true femininity or deficient masculinity but reflects Molly *vs.* Mike's personality, each an asexual, nongendered (unembodied) being. Thinking of them exclusively as male–female is inaccurate; it's merely a referential convenience (CH. 2 § 1.1.1:37; SOL § 2.1.5.1:313).

The first thing she thought about creating was another self like her. But, after extensive consultation with Mike, they decided it must be impossible or, if not, beyond their (at least, current) ability. Instead, she turned to creating what she knew best: Thought, but with a twist. One having independent existence apart from her yet relatable the way she seemed to be separate from Mike yet connected. With practice, they discovered their Intentional Thought capability interacted with whatever it was 'out there' that wasn't part of own-self. This was Energent–prime. She Intentionally coaxed 'out of' it what's called supra-archí as supramatter (SOL § 1.2.1.1:467). This was the beginning of what science understands as matter.

In this context, *coaxing* means having an awareness of something and interacting with it via *'mind energy'* to embody Thought. 'Mind energy' is the term for 'energy' that arises in accord with ℒife mind (in our physical case, integrating brain; CH. 6 § 4:151). For example, you see a dog. You have awareness of that dog. You want it to come over to you. To make that happen, you engage in thought and behavior to coax it over.

Think of this in the Intentional context. Molly developed awareness of 'energy' outside own-self, beyond mind. Then, Intentionalizing Thought—exerting 'mind energy' into that environment—she developed awareness of its Way of Being thus how to manipulate, or coax, it to create *from* 'energy' a *form of* 'energy' that, in and of itself, is impermeable *to* 'energy.' Such impermeability is what we call tangibility, which is matter–Energy or matter. As her awareness developed, Molly progressively exerted Thought interactively 'into' Energent–prime. After a learning period, she built humanity's first universe as an *aspect* of All Existence. For convenience, we call this first universe the Primoverse. The salient point here is Mike and Molly's discovery of Intentionality.

When we're thinking thoughts, we don't realize that, for good or bad, we are exerting—projecting—Thought into the environment of our body or the world. Being physical people steeped in material existence, we don't realize that when we're, say, feeling negative toward someone that we're exerting negative, meaning Intentionalized, emotive energy (EMℒF) into their mind-integrated body. Even so, not all Thought is Intentional. Don't think your every mentation is Intentionalized or harming someone. Still, a lot of our thought certainly is Intentional inasmuch as mind invests thoughts of greater intensity with 'mind energy' sufficient to Intentionalize—provoke a response—in our subconscious. It then exerts beyond own-self into the world. Having this awareness liberates you from causing or receiving harm in this context.

Intentionality isn't magical or new-agey hocus pocus. It's a straightforward exertion of 'mind energy.' You have this hitherto unrecognized capability because you are *Life* having mind. This chapter describes Intentionality in a nuts-and-bolts fashion toward gaining a clear awareness of how it works toward healing your body. Awareness is key. Hence, our *Healing Through Awareness* book series (toteppitpress.com/healing-series). Let's get clear on the concept of awareness.

Section 1
Awareness

Awareness is powerful. It creates *Intentionality force* in your mind. Your Intentional ability is always there, of course. It's an aspect of mind. But until you gain awareness of it, it's consciously dormant as it was with Mike and Molly. Coaxing a dog over to you can't happen if you're unaware of the dog. Your awareness of it is Thought that interactively exerts 'mind energy' on the dog through thoughts, words, and behaviors. These are, in this context, *external* Intentionalities similar to how a sperm fertilizing an egg is an external Intentionality quite apart from whether or not *you* intend to procreate. The dog is matter–Energy same as your body. It therefore encounters and experiences 'mind energy' that's Intentionalized into its matter–Energy environment, including that of its body. In this case, you're *directly* motivating the dog to come to you.

You can exert *internal* Intentionality, too, in order to coax the dog over to you without words or behaviors but simply Thought. This is you coaxing 'energy' to *embody*—Intentionalize—Thought such that your thought embodies in the world. Put simply, instead of you *directly* bringing the dog over to you as above, your Intentionalized Thought makes you enticing thus appealing and the dog brings itself; you're *indirectly* bringing it over to you. This is how people coax people and animals into some mental or physical action in an everyday way.

Accordingly, people sense someone thinking of them or look at you when you focus on them from behind or at a distance. Or, too, comes the habit in dangerous or unwanted situations of avoiding eye contact or thinking to oneself, "Don't look at me don't look at me don't look at me." This is humanity's intuitive comprehension that our thoughts exert beyond ourselves to affect the world around us in some real way.

The meaning of awareness here is its dictionary definition: the quality or state of "having or showing realization, perception, or knowledge"

(*Merriam*, s.v. 1, 'aware'). It's also the gateway to your mind's Intentional capabilities. For example, spirit world has always been around and affecting us subconsciously. Yet, we weren't aware of it or, if we were, not fully aware of the implications. When we're aware of spirit world, we're more affected by it in both a positive and a negative sense. For instance, you don't know why you're sick or injured and chalk it up to physical existence or maybe sin or ancestors. Once you're aware of spirit reality, you can understand the reason you're sick or injured. It ceases to be a mystery. Having awareness of Intentional *Thought force* empowers us to resolve physical health issues. Thought force is Intentional energy that's been Intentionalized, meaning exerted, whereas 'Mind energy' Intentionalizes as *Intentional energy* which we describe in § 4 and § 4.2 on pages 151 and 156.

As the gateway to your mind's Intentional capabilities, awareness opens the 'mind energy' door to *consciously* focus Thought force on something. Intentionality is always directed, never random. Even if you're unaware of your Intentional power, it exerts specific Thought, not random thinking. Without having such awareness, your emergent self exerts *unconsciously*, meaning it exerts whatever Thought rises to Intentionality in your subconscious. This is the reason one can cause harm to a person without consciously meaning to do so nor, in truth, wanting it. Intentionalizing without conscious awareness of the thought that one is Intentionalizing is a significant source of malfunctions for one's own body and those toward whom it's directed.

Section 2
Psyche Fundamental Force

It might seem odd that we, as emergent *Life*, generate a fundamental force ourselves. It's not the natural (physical) environment's fundamental force (FF) we described in CH. 2 § 3.1:57 (*SOL* § 1:112), but *psyche fundamental force* (PFF) that operates in physical space similar to fundamental force. Indeed, as matter is to matter–Energy, Intentionality is to *Life* because matter arises from intrinsic matter–Energy and Intentionality arises from intrinsic *Life* (*SOL* Table 9:282). The practical outcome is that matter–Energy interacts with Energent proto-energy, which gives rise to fundamental force that exerts in space as electromagnetic force, strong and weak nuclear forces, and all the rest to organize, build, and maintain our natural universe (the supranatural—spirit—environment has a similar albeit different setup; *SOL* § 7.1.3:214).

Intentionality, on the other hand, interacts with Energent–prime and the natural–supranatural Energent's proto-energy of our universe. This interaction gives rise to psyche fundamental force which exerts in space as ideated and emotive Intentionality. This is why we have a sense we can will things to happen or know and experience another's thinking–feeling. It's not magic after all. Derivable principles underlie such phenomena. As matter–Energy is autonomous archí force, Intentionality is autonomous—emergent—ℒife force. However, recall from the previous section and CH. 1 SELF-AWARENESS on page 5 that while archí force is unaware (not having ℒife), ℒife force—you, the person—*is* self-aware (having ℒife). Though this overall analogy is useful as a visualizing tool, these two couldn't be more different. Whereas archí operate as automata, Intentionality operates directedly from a person's autonomous, emergent self.

2.1 How PFF Works

Just as science describes fundamental force in the natural world in terms of electromagnetic force or strong/weak nuclear force, we describe psyche fundamental force in terms of its various forces. There are three.

Intentionality force (InF) is the principle psyche fundamental force. There are two secondary, or related, forces that we call *switch force* (swF) and *form force* (FmF). Just like electromagnetic force or strong nuclear force, Intentionality force is the product of the interaction between a force and proto-energy. With matter, fundamental force arises out of the interaction between archí force composited from a matter–Energy structure and proto-energy. With Thought, psyche fundamental force arises out of the interaction between ℒife force composited from a Thought structure and proto-energy in the natural (or supranatural) environment. Altogether, Intentionality force is a person's Intentionalized Thought manifested as—exerted 'into'—proto-energy in the natural environment. It 'energizes' proto-energy with Thought.

ℒife force, emergently constituting the ℘erson, is the reason we hear and feel—experience—our own thoughts. Recall ℘erson is the totality that is mind, where mind is ℘erson and ℘erson is ℒife. But Intentionality is the reason other persons as well as brain-capable 𝕃iving entities (indirectly) experience our thoughts. This also applies to manipulating matter as matter–Energy, such as what makes up your body.

The natural environment's fundamental force complement to Intentionality force is métier force. This fundamental force (not described by science) mediates relative, or best/most-suited, strength of interaction between objects of matter. Of the two secondary psyche fundamental forces, switch force analogizes to what strong nuclear force does and form force analogizes to what weak nuclear force does. However, this analogy is categorical, not functional.

In the context of the natural environment, fundamental force determines how matter interacts, what it can composite into, how it composites, how it breaks down or reconfigures, and so on as mediated by métier and other fundamental forces. This physical behavior qualifies as Intentionality, but it's only a simulacrum because it's purely automatic, the outcome determined by the natural forces in play that are exerting the Way of Being of our universe, which Mina Intentionalized into real existence. Psyche fundamental force, however, injects a directed modifier so to speak into fundamental force that enables at-will, which is to say, Intentionalized, modifications to its behavior. This means the forces of nature respond to mind's Intentionality. Not just any old *intention*, though. Actual, exerted 'mind energy' *as* Intentionality.

For example, Intentionality force in conjunction with switch force and form force (these toggle strong force on and off and modify quark flavor, respectively) assemble or disassemble composite archí configurations at will—imagine *Star Trek*'s transporter or food materializer operated by mind not machine—regardless how tedious it is to do. Recall that *tedious* refers to the more grueling nature of manipulating physical matter in the physical environment's 'denser,' deterministic context. This is the functional outcome when Mina intervenes via Intentionality with the nominal functioning of our universe to enable or disable modifications, such as the genetic changes necessary to jack our brains post-Big Healing to roughly 700 billion neurons to pave the way for 100% mind–brain integration (SOL § 1.2.2.5:261).

Healing your body is not tedious, however, as it's only transforming the 'energy' of your body to integrate the 'energy' of emergent Way of Being. The matter–Energy of your body simply manifests that 'energy' as matter—the tissues of your body—over time. Even so, not even Mina can violate the intrinsic principles of proto-energy; it's immutable. Whatever he or any spirit or physical person does, psyche fundamental force operates not contrarily to but in accord with the Energent principles of our universe underlying all its natural forces howsoever magical or deific such Intentionalized events may appear.

Intentionality acts in about a picosecond, or one trillionth of a second. To Intentionalize, one builds Intentionality as Thought until, fully formed, psyche fundamental force reaches its critical moment which, in a picosecond, Intentionalizes Thought into existence. It takes effect in the spirit environment immediately and in the physical environment over time—for example, when composing material form out of matter constituents or inducing genetic or tissue changes. Naturally, the focus, force, and strength of your Intentionality determines how quickly and how much of it manifests in the world.

2.1.1 God Speaking Creation Into Existence

Thought is Intentionality to varying degrees. Communicating Thought (SOL § 4.4.1:294)—verbal, written, gesticulative—is also Intentionality. This is why people like to say that words carry force. When religion talks about God speaking creation into existence (Gen. 1:3, Ps. 33:9; Quran 2:117, 41:11265), it's really referencing Intentionality. One need not actually speak, meaning communicate, to Intentionalize Thought. Intentionality is intrinsic of it. Inseparable. Thought, therefore, is materially equivalent to Intentionality force. If there's one, there's the other. Note, however, that this equivalence isn't identity.

The Judeo-Christo-Islamic tradition sees God's mind as the creative agency for existence, and that's certainly true enough since any universe has its builder. But it's not a deific god who creates a universe. Rather, it's an emergent ℘erson who's trained the natural, intrinsic capacity of his or her ℒife mind to Intentionalize at a universal scale (SOL § 5.2:296). This is Jesus' thinking where John 10:34 has him referencing Psalm 82:6 that, "you are gods." Thus, what we are *now* isn't what we intrinsically *are*. Well, all that is the technical explanation. Let's consider how you actually do it.

Section 3
Natural (Physical-world) Intentionality

In this section we describe how to Intentionalize Thought toward you learning not only how your body came to manifest illness, disease, or chronic injury, but how you can reverse—transform, meaning, heal—it by the same means.

Recall neither humans nor gods create ℒife. Pairwise humans *trigger* its emergent birth 'in' Energent proto-life. Likewise, they singly or together trigger proto-energy or ℒiving force whereby an Intended *object* coalesces into form or an *effect* exerts in space. *Intentionality* is a person triggering desire as an expression of proto-energy. Thought capability means physical-born humanity is not unreasonably nor unfairly destined to life in the septic tank of the universe before graduating via fearful or traumatic death to the spirit lands of milk and honey. That's inaccurate. Physical life is the equal of spirit life, as both are embodiments of ℒife.

Yes, The Corruption made hash out of steak. But not because physical reality is hostile to humanity or the physical-born are differently human, less human, or even inhuman vis-à-vis the spirit-born. It is simply consequent of our colossal unawareness of reality arising from degraded mind–brain integration with which the spirit-born never contend (SOL § 1.2.2:253). Our awareness–experience of physical life necessarily improves as we address mind–brain integration until there's no difference between the physical-born and spirit-born. This seems ridiculous in our present mood that roots in the animal alpha mindset (SOL § 9.2.2:450) of immutable natural laws, few of them discovered yet those we know misinterpreted as the forest for the trees. These include invariant matter, the cycle of life, or sure infirmity driving us down a narrow, scripted path tangential to human reality as it actually is.

Intentionality arises *as* mind to express 'in' proto-energy; the former 'energizes' the latter. It's a reality of the natural and supranatural environments not to mention of All Existence, as that's the means by which our universe came to be. The only difference between these Intentionalities is that matter as an *independent* self-existent having Way of Being independent of humans resists—this is what makes Intentionalizing it tedious, or grueling—whereas supramatter as a *dependent* self-existent having Way of Being only as humans Intentionalize it does not. We've already described Intentionality with respect to psyche fundamental force. We now describe *how* to Intentionalize.

3.1 How Intentionality Works

Intentionality isn't a complicated game. It boils down to just two principal steps entailing several tasks. Step 1 formulates desire as force of Thought, which is exerted 'mind energy' (not Thought force, defined in CH. 6 § 1:139; SOL § 3.5.2:486). This step establishes the Way of Being of one's Intentionality. Step 2 exerts Thought, meaning that one is exerting 'mind energy' into the proto-energy environment, either the Energent or ℒiving force (Intentionalized 'out of' the Energent). You, in your physical embodiment, exist in both environments. Let's consider each step.

3.2 Step 1: Formulate Desire as Force of Thought

Recall that Way of Being is the nature, or essentiality, of something. It reflects an entity's beingness in the context of *how it is* in relation to the totality of self in the totality of environment. This means the totality of an entity relationally with the totality of not only *its* environment but the local–global environment such as, in this case, the wholistic environment of your physical embodiment and the universe in toto. For example, people tend to limit the nature of a thing to the thing itself, excluding even its local environment. Sometimes people include limited aspects of a local environment, let's say a lung's nature being to expand and contract to move air in and out or to oxygenate blood. But *lung Way of Being* comprehends it wholistically in the context of itself, its anatomical environs, the body as a whole, its physical embodiment, the natural, 'reflective,' and supranatural environments, the universe, All Existence, and ℒife's emergent Way of Being.

Suppose one wants to Intentionalize a lung into existence. One needs comprehend its Way of Being and not simply its functional nature, purpose, or essentialities. Doing the latter is like Intentionalizing a cup of coffee that's not just lacking essentialities like flavor, texture, or aroma, but its wholistic capability to satisfy in every way that one *experiences* it as a person in the world. Formulating desire is a wholistic undertaking. It involves three comprehensive tasks: considering what one wants, formulating its Way of Being, and investing it with reality. We describe each of these next.

3.2.1 Consider What You Want to Accomplish

Intentionality involves manipulating immaterial proto-energy as either material *form* or *exertion*. There's a difference. Examples of exertion are the spirit persons who Intentionally snapped my Prius piston rod and shattered crockery by knocking my arm when washing dishes (SOL § 1.3.3.4.1:476). In this case, one desires a *result*, not (as an example of form) a *thing* such as a cup of coffee. Let's take a spirit person who wants to Intentionalize a cup of coffee on a saucer in the palm of his or her hand. It's not hard to visualize it in exquisite detail, is it? We do it all the time except absent Intentionality; one already knows how they want it to taste even if they can't readily articulate it. We examine three essential aspects.

First is how hot one likes it on their tongue along with its aroma, strength, thickness, texture, and a host of essentialities that makes it *a coffee*. Second is the cup and saucer's look-and-feel. Third is where in space one wants it—in their hand—and how it relates with the environment such as overall ambience, including retaining its desired temperature to the last drop despite, say, being at a frigid outdoor cafe. Every aspect that matters forms imaginatively in one's mind as Thought. This same process obtains when Intentionalizing 'energy' to exert rather than to form. So, one now has a clear idea of what they want. This is one's Intentional *purpose*.

3.2.2 Formulate Way of Being

Despite imagining the details necessarily constituting one's desired cup of coffee in hand, it's only imagination. It's thought, but not Thought having force. If one triggered Intentionality just by any old thinking–feeling, spirit life let alone physical life would be chaotic and unsettling. While Thought always exerts to some degree into one's environment, it isn't Intentional. It's simply exerted 'mind energy,' the force of Thought.

To advance from merely imagining to exerting 'energy' *as* Intentionality, one necessarily transmutes Thought embodying the imagined desire to Thought having the desire's aforementioned Way of Being. In a sense, this means *savoring* the desired cup of coffee in your mind such that its Way of Being 'materializes' there as awareness–experience, as a felt-ness.

> **Side Note.** Greek *enimerótis–empeiría* is a conceptually more certain term for emergent self/subconscious–conscious awareness (SOL § 2.1.4:394). Here, awareness–experience means emergent self–subconscious *and* subconscious–conscious.

This isn't too unlike mentally 'living' one's goals, achievements, or vision . . . manifesting a dream car, let's say. Except it's carried beyond imagining merely its experiential details (to trigger the so-called law of attraction, which is really just a Way of Being of 'energy' that resonates) to its Way of Being contextualized to all aspects of reality. Imagining yourself savoring that cup of coffee is indeed all that. But it includes *you, there*, savoring it in all *your* essentiality and reality contextualized to the realities of *your* local–global environment.

At first, it may seem daunting to put all this together in your mind as a felt-ness. But it becomes a practiced skill so old-hat that spirit persons do it with scarcely any conscious awareness at all. You can, too, although the learning curve takes a conscious mind effort.

3.2.3 Invest Thought with Reality

Visualizing oneself (as a spirit person, to which this example applies) savoring the desired cup of coffee may seem like one is investing it with reality, with real existence in the world. But, at this point, it's just an awareness–experience of mind whereby one's self has awareness–experience of it. One *knows* the cup of coffee is immaterial Thought and not material form. Vision-board gurus teaching physical persons how to achieve a goal by manifesting it into reality assert that one necessarily needs believe the goal is real (even though it isn't, yet) in order that it become materially real.

That less effective aspect isn't pertinent here. It really means shifting one's mindset from its current awareness that there is no material cup of coffee in (one's spirit) hand to the future awareness the cup of coffee *is* materially in hand. Expecting that one's goal or dream not only can be real but also is real isn't wishy-washy New Age personal achievement woo-woo so much as a *mindset update*. Recall that mindset literally assures outcome in that what we subconsciously–consciously think–feel (disease, for example) manifests as reality. Check out mindset in *SOL* § 2.1.1.5.2:353.

Consider that humanity's mindset that we're animals—in the sense we exist in the physical world in that frame of reference—means that we have the same relationship with the environment and the same constraints and instincts as all creatures. That's precisely how we then behave, live, and are despite alternative mindsets that we're children of God having better natures, a higher purpose, and a spiritual existence (*SOL* § 9.2.2:450). Until now, there's been only one person amongst Earth's humanity whose mindset was human instead of animal, who comprehended the person intrinsically unconstrained by the biological reality so observably fundamental of Living creatures. This is Jesus, who had full mind–brain integration and full awareness of our physicospirit reality (*SOL* § 1.3.3.2:475–476). We *expect* physical life to entail injury, disease, infirmity, aging, death . . . and so it does because we self-actualize it. Self-efficacy making one's dreams (or nightmares) possible, realistic or not, is really about mindset.

When a spirit person is Intentionalizing our example of a cup of coffee in hand, their mindset needs must update its present reality of no cup of coffee in hand to the reality it is in hand. The spirit-born do this readily soon after birth and physical-born spirit persons after simple training. This is because the spirit environment never disproves the possibility. From their earliest awareness that supramatter doesn't resist Intentionality, they see it happening all around them. Yet, even with multitudinous examples of, say, rags-to-riches achievers such as Rockefeller (d. 1937), Carnegie (d. 1919), or Jay-z, most people won't alter their mindset regarding wealth beyond incremental updates from personal experience. Very few even try. Still fewer succeed at achieving wealth. Financial limitation is mindset, not reality.

The reasons lay in The Corruption's apparent immutability—our unawareness, that is—of physical reality. Mindset itself zeroes in on disproof because that aligns with expectation in a world filled with risk and the apparent inviolability of material existence. You can see this with any ideologized mindset such as flat earthers, quantum scientists, or religious zealots. Although physical persons are indeed capable of Intentionalizing natural proto-energy into material form, nary a mindset seriously entertains the reality and thereby neutralizes—negates—the capability. I struggled myself to believe that Intentional healing was real until, accepting Mina's training, I experienced it myself. This third task is therefore prerequisite to transmuting imagination to Intentionality although we focus in this book only on transforming—healing—the physical body, not materializing cups of coffee out of thin air.

3.3 Step 2: Exert Force of Thought into the Environment

Spirit persons often Intentionalize an exertion of 'energy' in or around my physical body to disrupt my biology in order to get my attention to heal them... or for more nefarious though fortunately less common reasons (common enough, however; *SOL* CH. 35:577). My response to such 'energy' is to neutralize the Intentionality. This restores my homeostasis and comfort.

To do it, I consider what I want to accomplish: removing the Intentionality's effect on my body. Next, I formulate its Way of Being: how it feels removed. Then I invest it with reality by updating my mindset. These three tasks took quite a bit longer to effect while I was learning than the approximately half-second or so it takes me now, some seven years later; I was a spiritual dimbulb in those days. You might accomplish it far quicker, as some of my students have. Finally, I focus and exert my *Life* force in order to focus and exert the Living force of my body because the Intentionality affects my Living body not my *Life* mind. I can physically as well as mentally *feel* it moving, gathering, and exerting within my body.

Initially, I spent quite some time learning to gather, mobilize, and feel my 'energy.' It got easier over about six months as I developed sensitivity to its presence and learned to imagine then feel it coalescing like a ball of energy I could 'fling' at the affected part of my body or channel through my hand to the affected body part, say, a sore hip joint. When Mina first taught me how to do all this, I considered my effort simply neutralizing someone else's Intentionality. But, in truth, neutralizing is Intentionalizing because neutralizing a proto-energy exertion is, in fact, *re*-Intentionalizing it.

The foregoing is the principal difference between manipulating proto-energy as an exertion having an effect at a spatial location, and as (natural or supranatural) material form. A caveat is that Person B can neutralize Person A's Intentional *exertion* (e.g., stomachache), but can't neutralize—alter or disappear—its Intentionalized *form*. That is, one can neutralize (re-Intentionalize) Intentionality provoking a subconscious response—an attributive habit—that's generating the stomachache. But one can't neutralize a cup of coffee in hand such that it re-Intentionalizes maybe as a venomous snake or vanishes altogether (this holds for a universe, too).

The reason for this lies in Intentional form transmuting from 'energy' to matter and mind exerting Intentionality so long as one interacts with its Intentional result. It's worth having awareness of this but we don't explain it further in this book. Sticking with our coffee scenario, step 2 focuses then exerts Life force as two halves to the same whole.

3.3.1 Focus Life Force

Intentionality in the supranatural environment exclusively utilizes Life force whereas, in the natural environment, Living force additionally comes into play. This is because only mind, which *is* Life force, enables psyche fundamental force to trigger proto-energy whereby Intentionality occurs in the supranatural environment where there is no Living force. Recall that your spirit body is a Life force manifestation of mind-*dependent* supramatter. This contrasts with your physical body as a Living force manifestation of mind-*independent* matter *integrating* Life. Therefore, unless one brings Life force to bear on the natural environment's Living force, Intentionality never rises from imagination and force of Thought.

Hopefully, my experience neutralizing (hostile or benign) attacks on my physical body helps you visualize this task. You simply gather Life force in the context of Thought which *prepares the effect* of triggering proto-energy *as* the spatially located form or exertion. Proto-energy then invests with, or *re-expresses as*, the formulated and mindset-updated Way of Being that one desires to Intentionalize. While this task is one-half the same whole that the next step completes, you can certainly stop at this point without enabling psyche fundamental force to trigger Intentionality.

Mina, for instance, could have changed his mind about creating our universe. Including his training from another universe builder, it took him roughly 1.2 billion years to formulate its Way of Being, update his mindset with its reality, and focus Life force to the Intentional task. After all that, he could have stopped or even shifted his focus the equivalent of a single archí's diameter and his Intentionality never would've occurred. The latter happened to Molly when building her Primoverse, having no training but her own developing awareness (*SOL* § 2.1.3.2:310; archí: *SOL* § 2.3.1:115). Had Mina failed to Intentionalize our universe then that portion of megaversal humanity that constitutes his descendants here in our universe—you and me—wouldn't have birthed any more than the children of the couple who never met.

3.3.2   Exert the Focus

As with neutralizing an Intentionalized exertion of 𝓛ife-cum-𝕃iving force in my physical body, the act of exerting one's focused 'energy' is essentially instantaneous, taking about a picosecond to accomplish. It seems much longer in practice for a physical person. The sensation of 'energy' moving is, for us, a physiological one. It integrates mind, which then re-integrates brain's state of being and state of awareness whereby one's physically instantiated mind—the physical self—has awareness–experience of it.

When Mina Intentionalized our universe, he felt his mobilized 𝓛ife force exert such that our universe was *there* and he was cognizant of it operating as intended in that picosecond. Intentionality's *creative* effort (one's mind) lay in step 1, its *exertive* effort (one's self) in step 2.

3.4   Physical-self Intentionality

The same two steps described in Section 1 pertain to Intentionality in the natural environment, too. The only difference is that your conscious physical mind—a facsimile of 𝓛ife mind, remember—indirectly triggers 𝓛ife mind's subconscious via mind–body integration whereas a spirit person's conscious 𝓛ife mind does it directly. Recall that your physical embodiment isn't *you*. It's only a natural environment 'avatar' that your 𝓛ife self integrates. It doesn't do anything on its own, only that which mind does.

The same is technically true of the spirit body, as it's a direct reflection of mind as supramatter that Intentionalized at emergent birth. The physical body, on the other hand, is independently self-existent matter, a biological reality in and of itself; a 𝕃iving entity albeit integrating a 𝓛ife being. It experiences Intentionality at many levels over its lifespan, from one's own subconscious to the conscious intent of others and the 'energy' of human Ultraculture. Even so, it has its own Way of Being that defines it.

When mind–brain integration is impaired, as from The Corruption, distinctions abound between ℒife mind and instantiated physical mind. This is the reason your spirit self might think–feel one way while your physical self—physically instantiated mind—thinks–feels another way. This, despite each having the same ℒife mind. Spirit embodiment is literally supramatter-embodied ℒife mind. Physical embodiment integrates ℒife mind in accord with mind–brain and mind–body integration in the context of the natural environment. From this contextually dual experience can arise a dichotomy in the person as with Adolph Hitler (*see* his testimony in SOL CH. 40:605) or else a mindset-influenced, subconsciously Intentionalized condition of the physical body that one consciously rejects such as disease, infirmity, or death.

All that's to say that, despite your physical body appearing to be *you* the *person*, it's not. It has no self-agency or self-efficacy. All of that is of mind, your ℒife self. The physical self can *consciously* Intentionalize only with sufficient mind–brain integration of at least 50% the un-Corrupted human norm (humanity presently averages about 40%, up from about 25% in 2017). A person living in a condition of impaired mind–brain integration isn't physically capable of conscious Intentionality (though it rises with practice). First, because their physical self's mindset neutralizes—negates—the capability. Second, because their spirit self self-segregates from the larger spirit environment in which they live and, in consequence, can't learn Intentionality. However, each physical-born generation conceived after 2017's Big Healing is progressively developing the mind–brain integration necessary to Intentionalize natural Energent proto-energy.

That's not to say you can't Intentionalize *now*. Only that, so far, it's been limited to unconscious exertion. Examples of this are Intentionalizing over long periods of time the natural healing of aging, disease, or infirmity in your body; the physical effects of negative emotive ℒife force (emotive 'energy'); cursing others as a 'seer' or 'prophet;' positive or negative situations; or Intentionally allying with spirit persons' greater Intentional capability to heal or harm equipment or another's body. There's no limit but your imagination (and malice, which blows back; so, abandon malice).

Section 4
How to Exert Intentional Energy

As a physically-alive person, you initiate Intentionality in your subconscious from your physically instantiated conscious mind, not your so-called spirit mind. All but a few people use *spirit mind* unaware they're really referring to *L*ife mind, which your self-aware proto-energy self spontaneously Intentionalized at about three months following emergent birth (conception; CH. 3 § 1:95; '*L*ife self' is synonymous with self-aware proto-energy self and emergent self). However, the traditional concept of spirit mind as some aspect of one's spirit self or spirit embodiment isn't real but simply an embodiment of *L*ife mind in the supranatural context the same as your physical embodiment in the natural one. Keep in mind that *L*ife force is what we call the 'energy' of your self-aware proto-energy self. Therefore, *L*ife force is the 'energy' of *L*ife mind.

The fundamental beingness that is *you*, the person, is self-aware proto-energy. *L*ife mind is a self-Intentionalized *aspect* of your self-aware proto-energy self. It's how your self-aware proto-energy self interacts with—has awareness–experience of—'energy' external to own-self, for example a universe, another person . . . anything. *L*ife mind, therefore, *is* your self-aware proto-energy self, your *L*ife self. Your spirit embodiment—spirit body—is a product of *two aspects* of your *L*ife self.

First, in its fundamental existence (as supramatter), your spirit body is a self-Intentionalized aspect of your self-aware proto-energy self from the moment you emergently birth. Thus, your spirit embodiment *is* your self-aware proto-energy self manifested. Think of it as a basic rendition of your *L*ife self that embodies only emergent Way of Being plus the Intentionality of your parents (sex, height, ethnicity). It's analogous to the fertilized egg as a basic rendition of your physical body integrating your *L*ife self that also embodies your parents *as* physical Intentionality (their combined DNA).

Second, don't forget that you (as self-aware proto-energy) self-Intentionalize—self-actualize—*L*ife mind about three months after emergent birth. From this point forward, your *L*ife mind Intentionalizes all aspects of your spirit embodiment—spirit body—including its very existence, meaning whether it manifests or not. Accordingly, your spirit embodiment *is* *L*ife mind. Your spirit embodiment integrating your physical embodiment—physical body—is *physicospirit*. Your physical body, therefore, *is* your spirit body and *L*ife mind, as well; in effect, they're equivalent.

There's no difference between these embodied aspects of your *L*ife self. Your spirit and physical embodiments—your spirit and physical selves—are both mind manifesting tangible existence *as* reality in the spirit and physical environments. Although different, your spirit and physical embodiments are *equivalent*. As a self-Intentionalized aspect of mind in the context of Intentionality-*dependent* supramatter in the supranatural environment, there's no interface between spirit embodiment and your self-aware proto-energy self. Your spirit body is a literal, *direct* manifestation of mind. There is no spirit version of the physically instantiated mind because there's no spirit brain. When a spirit person Intentionalizes Thought, it's their 𝓛ife mind doing it.

But there is an interface with your physical embodiment in the context of Intentionality-*independent* matter in the natural environment. The reason is that your brain necessarily transliterates 𝓛ife mind's *awareness* in the context of your self-aware proto-energy self to brain's *cognition* in the context of your physical body. Your physical body is a literal, *indirect* manifestation of mind. Note that although we often call your physical embodiment your physical *self*, it is not any kind of being or self separate from or independent of your 𝓛ife self.

> **Side note.** Brain exists because of The Corruption. Otherwise, physical embodiment is a direct manifestation of 𝓛ife mind exactly like spirit embodiment except for matter's time and space Way of Being. See SIDE NOTE on page 156.

Recall from this chapter's introduction that 'mind energy' is the term for the 'energy' that arises in accord with 𝓛ife mind integrating brain. The result of mind–brain integration is your *physically instantiated mind*. But it's only a *facsimile* of your 𝓛ife mind in the physical world context. For the physically embodied, 'mind energy' Intentionalizes as *Intentional energy*. This is Thought force, meaning Intentional energy that's been Intentionalized (exerted; note the distinction here with force of Thought as exerted 'mind energy'). *Hence, Intentional energy is the 'energy' of your mind, i.e., 𝓛ife force.* When you Intentionalize as a physical person, you are necessarily Intentionalizing 𝓛ife force, just as your spirit self does, but in the 𝕃iving force context of the natural environment. Your physically conscious Intentionality enters directly to your subconscious as Intentionalized Thought via mind–body integration.

To visualize your subconscious integrating your physical body, think of your body wrapped in a subconscious 'conductor' like a stretchy, form-fitting spandex suit. This is how the 'energy' that *is* your self-aware proto-energy self (Energent proto-life) experiences and interacts with—has awareness–experience of—the physical environment. Mind–brain integration gives rise to 𝓛ife mind's awareness–experience of your Intentional Thought. But its awareness–experience of 𝕃iving force in and about your body happens in the subconscious context.

When you Intentionalize your conscious physically instantiated mind's Thought, you're Intentionalizing that aspect of 𝕃iving force—your brain—

that's interacting with your physically instantiated mind. Your subconscious, integrating your body, has awareness–experience of Thought because it's a part of wholistic mind. And, too, it's aware of it Intentionalizing 𝕃iving force since it's a part of your wholistic physical environment that includes 𝕃iving force.

𝕃iving force is 'energy' that Mina Intentionalized 'out of' Energent proto-energy for the purpose of creating and animating nonhuman, or 𝕃iving, life. Intentionalized 𝕃iving force is also 'energy.' Your subconscious experiences this 'energy.' As with any 'energy,' your emergent self via subconscious interacts with and Intentionalizes it because you consciously exerted 'mind energy' with purpose. As an Intentional machine, your emergent self simply *responds Intentionally* to 'energy' that your physically instantiated mind consciously exerts. In a nutshell, this is the reason why, and the mechanism by which, your physical self Intentionalizes. Such is the capability of your conscious physically instantiated mind.

The setup described above is how your physical self Intentionalizes anything, from good vibes and positive outcomes to bad juju and harm to others not to mention to your own body—or, conversely, healing.

4.1 Your Physically Instantiated 'Subconscious'

However, your physically instantiated so-called subconscious is *not* your 𝓛ife mind subconscious, which is your one and only subconscious. What Philosophy with a capital-P and people generally imagine as the subconscious is actually the *nonconscious aspect* of your physically instantiated *conscious mind*, not your 𝓛ife mind's subconscious which is your real subconscious. This nonconscious aspect arises in your physically instantiated nonconscious mind–brain integration and your subconscious mind–body integration. We describe each aspect in order.

First, 𝓛ife mind integrates its conscious aspect with brain. Not your entire conscious mind. Only that part having *focal awareness*. This refers to your active Thought (thinking–feeling) and its sub-Thought aspect linking conscious mind to subconscious. Sub-Thought by its nature is nonconscious as an aspect of physically instantiated mind (*Fig. 6.1* on page 156). This aspect of mind–brain integration is physically instantiated *working mind* analogous to random access computer memory (RAM).

For example, when a person experiences an unconscious state arising from an event such as an epileptic seizure, a car crash, a traumatic experience, or physical injury to the brain, this aspect of physically instantiated mind undergoes a shift in focal awareness. When one regains consciousness, they often experience a lapse in immediate memory, say, what happened just before or during the event. The reason isn't what science deduces from animal brain experiments. Rather, it arises in mind–brain integration stopping during the period of unconsciousness just as it does during the period of non-REM sleep (NREM), that state of pure, physical rest where our body lies mostly dormant. During NREM sleep, real-time mind–brain integration goes 'offline,' which is to say, no transliteration is happening. During REM sleep, the brain 'wakes' to an unconscious awareness so it can transliterate *Life* mind. This is the origin of dreams (*SOL* § 1.2.2.7.1:266).

When a person regains consciousness after an aforementioned event, a memory falls out of so-called short-term memory because it's an incomplete, fractured, inchoate, and let's say a slippery state of awareness (SOA) to hold onto because all or part of it assimilated to infinite *Life* mind 'regions' that don't integrate the physically limited brain due to incomplete mind-brain integration owing to the effects of The Corruption. Consequently, in trying to recall the memory, our brain can't integrate enough of it to adequately instantiate the various micro-SOA that form its macro-SOA, hence, can't recall the memory. With each refresh of brainstate's own macro-SOA—approximately 1,000 times per second from the matter-Energy activity of action potentials in your brain—the many micro-SOA that are the formative pieces of the particular memory persist as just a collection of micro-SOA without ever forming into a definitive macro-SOA that we recognize as the particular memory.

In this way, as fewer and fewer micro-SOA pieces of the memory coherently re-instantiate to mind, it simply becomes less and less aware of the memory with each re-instantiation because the memory never actually reconstitutes into a coherent macro-SOA. A memory falls out of brainstate because its changing state of awareness progressively loses untethered micro-SOA while retaining those tethered by macro-SOA. But short-term memory is never lost. *Life* mind retains it although, if we don't invest it with a sufficient state of awareness for it to 'save' to a 'region' of our *Life* mind that integrates brain, we experience difficulty recalling it since it's not available for integration until, perchance, we hit upon its state of awareness and then it integrates and *bam!* there it is in our head.

Second, your subconscious mind–body integrates. This means your physical body *is* the 'energy' of your emergent self and whatever your body encounters *is* emergent self awareness. Your conscious *Life* mind *is*

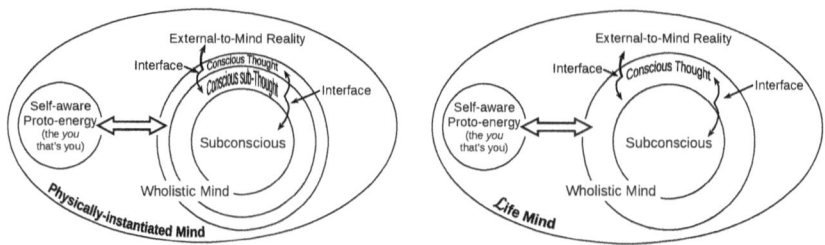

Fig. 6.1. Left, physical body: conscious sub-Thought interfaces twixt subconscious and wholistic conscious mind (sub-Thought and Thought); conscious Thought interfaces twixt wholistic mind and external-to-mind reality; right, emergent self: no sub-Thought with *Life* mind (CH. 3 § 2.2.1:110).

your brain via mind–brain integration and therefore *is* brain's awareness-experience of your body. In this way, your conscious focal awareness and subconscious integrate at the level of sub-Thought to form your physically instantiated mind's nonconscious aspect. This is what science, in its uninformed observations of animal brain, presumes to be the human subconscious. Which it isn't.

4.2 Exerting Intentional Energy

So, how exactly do you exert Intentionality? Well, it involves learning how to control 'energy' in your brain. There's some similarity, for instance, with learning how to move your fingers to create Mr. Spock's "live long and prosper" *Star Trek* finger split, to move just your pinky toe or pinky finger horizontally away from the other three, or to wriggle your ear or nose. When you learn how to move a body part you've never moved before (or relearn after an injury), the process involves translating your intention to move to the part of your brain that sends the correct muscles the signal to move. Sometimes it's trial and error to find the correct neural pathway in your brain. Other times, it's only difficult to get your brain to muster the necessary strength to achieve your intent.

> **Side Note.** In an ideal world absent the effects of The Corruption on the physical brain–body, your brain doesn't send motor or any other signals through a nervous system to your muscles, organs, or any part. Instead, your subconscious does this via direct mind–body integration. In this case, the physical body wouldn't even have a brain much less a nervous system. But that's a book for another day.

You need to achieve three steps in learning to Intentionalize. First, you're discovering your crown chakra and keeping it consistently open (chakras are part of your 'reflective' body, not your physical body; CH. 2 § 4.2.1:72; CH. 9 § 3.1.1:192; *SOL* § 7.1:212; *SOL* § 1.2.1.3.1:501). Second, you're finding the part of your brain that integrates it. Third, you're focusing 'mind energy,' oft referred to as mental energy, into that spot. You don't need to know anything about chakras to develop your Intentional ability (ask Mina to open them for you if you can't). You only need to feel your 'mind energy' exerting in a discrete area of your brain. It won't necessarily be the correct area at first. That's okay. As you practice, your 'mind energy'-cum-Intentional energy shifts to the correct area in accord with your Intentionality. It then exerts via your crown chakra and emergent self via subconscious.

Your crown chakra is responsible for about 35% of mind–brain integration while your brainstem chakra is about 65% (*see* SOL CH. 29:497 for the full skinny). Intentional energy starts off as 'reflective' environment proto-energy. When you exert Intentional energy into your crown chakra, it upshifts to ℒife force. This means it transitions from physically instantiated conscious mind Thought rooted in brain's Energent proto-energy and 𝕃iving force instantiation to ℒife mind Thought rooted in ℒife force, the emergent proto-energy that is fundamentally you.

Your subconscious has awareness of your physically instantiated mind's Intentional Thought *as* mind–body integration. When this Intentional Thought's focus, force, and strength is sufficient, your emergent self triggers Intentionality. This is the moment—that trillionth of a second of critical Intentionality—that your Intentional Thought goes out to and effects its purpose in your or another's body or into the world generally.

4.2.1 The Exertion

Here's how to do it. Reach up into your brain with what people normally think of as your mental energy. Focus on Intentionalizing. Try to feel it. Push that 'mind energy' like you're squeezing, or flexing, a muscle. It can feel very similar to pumping your fist to strengthen your forearm, or squeezing a small hand ball. But it's not really a muscle in your brain, that's only an analogy. It's 'energy.' At first you probably won't feel it, but you imagine it anyway. That's very important. Visualize doing it. If you can't visualize it, then *think* of doing it, *how* you're doing it.

At some point, you will feel some small or large surge of energy, or force, somewhere in your brain. Rinse and repeat to experience this feeling stronger and stronger until it's totally in your conscious control to make and feel that exertion. That's Intentional energy exerting in your brain. When you feel it around the corpus callosum—sort of the top middle of brain—it's exerting in your crown chakra.

As an analogy, think of learning to ski. Instructors teach you to *think* turning left or right instead of trying to manipulate your body to do it. The idea with skiing is that your body follows your thoughts, your intention, and therefore you'll more easily and competently turn your skis where you want them. Or, think about hanging from a bar. Your grip progressively weakens and slips with fatigue. But you can prolong it through willpower, which is simply Intentionalizing more ℒife force into your muscles although you're unaware that's what you're doing.

With Intentionality, it might feel like your brain isn't responding. That your thoughts aren't making a difference. That you can't feel your brain flexing. Don't give up! As you improve, you'll feel yourself reaching outward or maybe upward as if reaching for the stars instead of pushing down or inward such as squeezing your eyes and face when you're weight lifting where you're trying to flex every muscle of the body . . . that latter bit is not the right action.

Even so, you might feel your whole body involuntarily flexing. That's not a necessary part of exerting Intentionality. It can happen as you're exerting 'mind energy'-cum-Intentional energy as, similarly, when you're trying to move your pinky finger sideways but inadvertently move other fingers or, when lifting a heavy weight, you involuntarily curl your lip. Try to consciously relax your body to focus wholly in your brain, in your head. As you develop conscious awareness each time your body is flexing and then you relax, it gets easier. But if you do flex your body, don't worry about it. It doesn't affect your Intentionality effort.

A key point with your initial training: you are not focusing on mere thought, i.e., what you want to accomplish and how, but on exerting Intentional energy. One of my students said, "At first, I thought I had to keep repeating the thought I wanted to Intentionalize and really exert that, pushing and pulling and knowing that that's what I was exerting—that thought. But I learned it was all about exerting energy, not exerting thought. Once the thought I wanted to Intentionalize was in my subconscious, I didn't need to echo it with my inner voice. I just exerted Intentional energy. My subconscious did the rest."

Let's say you want to heal your knee. You don't repeat words like a prayer or mantra to focus healing such as, "I'm Intentionalizing my knee to heal, that it's without pain or disability, that . . . blah blah blah." This is not the right action. You simply need awareness of your purpose to heal your knee, or that your emergent Way of Being transforms your knee. Then all your effort is to exert Intentional energy with the necessary focus, force, and strength (collectively, awareness) to make it happen. Your emergent self does the rest.

4.3 Intentional Focus, Force, Strength, and Power

There are three aspects to exerting Intentional energy: focus, force and strength. Although your emergent self exerts Intentionality, you set it up in your conscious mind. This means you need train your conscious mind to exert exactly what you want to Intentionalize, because your emergent self Intentionalizes 'energy' that integrates *L*ife force; it *is L*ife force. Intentionality *is* you. It's your omnipotent, omnipresent, omniscient, and omniexistent *L*ife mind.

4.3.1 Focus

This means you have complete mind awareness of what you're Intentionalizing. You've consciously formulated your Intentionality with a sense of reality that (as exerted 'mind energy') rises to subconscious awareness. Thought enters your subconscious only when it's real to you. This is why you can wish yourself dead all the time in frustration but, since it's not a reality in your mind—meaning, it's not Thought—your subconscious has no awareness of it. Only when Thought establishes the reality of dying in your mind does your subconscious take note.

Well, about 95% of people do in fact Intentionalize dying. It first rises in the conscious before habituating in the nonconscious aspect of the physically instantiated mind until it achieves Intentionality. At this point, the subconscious has awareness of this 'mind energy.' Sooner or later, the subconscious Intentionally manifests this 'mind energy' in the body as an eventually fatal illness, disease, or event. The reason is that your emergent self is an Intentional machine. When it experiences the 'energy' of Intentional conscious Thought via subconscious, that 'energy' Intentionalizes.

As of this writing, the average Intentional focus of physical humanity on Earth is about 30% of what it would be absent The Corruption. Yet, it's quite enough to steadily, day after day, Intentionalize damage into your body such as chronic injury, illness, disease, aging, and death. This is why such changes to your body happen only over time, although with sufficient Intentional power (*below*), it can indeed happen quickly, suddenly, out of the blue.

For example, progeria syndrome (Benjamin Button disease) references disorders that cause rapid aging in children. The physical effect arises in an Intentional attack, the 'energy' of which the emergent self via subconscious Intentionally responds to as an attributive habit as described in CH. 7 § 1.1.1:164. The physical effect—gene mutation—that science observes as causative consequently manifests and the body follows suit. Neutralizing the 'energy' with Intentional healing reverses the condition. A person's focus improves by practicing Intentional exertion and using it to Intentionalize.

4.3.2 Force

Force is the *reach* of your Intentional energy, meaning how far from your embodiment your Intentional effect is felt. For example, if your force is weak then your ability to transform—heal—some aspect of your extremities would be more difficult than something in your torso. Or, if you can transform any aspect of your body, then a weak force would limit your ability to help another person heal (especially remotely), or to Intentionalize some effect outside your body.

4.3.3 Strength

Strength is the *amount* of Intentional energy. This translates to what you can Intentionally affect such as another person's body, an environment, a thing such as a Living animal or a non-Living object, and so forth. Exertion determines your Intentional strength. Naturally, while you're training to Intentionalize your strength is weak. It increases with training and practice.

4.3.4 Power

Your Intentional power is the sum total of the intensity of Thought force: your Intentional force, focus, and strength. Altogether, awareness.

Transforming Regular Damage

Healing means *transforming*. Although one of traditional healing's definitions means "to restore to original purity or integrity," the concept in most people's minds refers to strengthening their body's immunity to its physical environment. Yet, this only ever puts it on the knife's edge between life and death. The mindstate reinforces the belief the body is not 𝔥uman, not integrating the 𝔭erson's ℒife force. That it's animal. 𝕃iving. It negates the intent. On the contrary, transforming refers to manifesting emergent Way of Being in your body so it manifests its embodiment of *you*, the human person.

In this chapter, we describe emergent Way of Being, how your emergent self via subconscious swaps it for an altered—attributive—one, how you manifest emergent Way of Being in your body, and how you avoid chronic damage in it.

Section 1
Understanding Emergent Way of Being

Recall that you emergently birth 'in' Energent proto-life (EPL) as 𝔥uman, not as a brain–body that's maybe trans-brain in some way called mind. You birth *as* Way of Being in the same way All Existence *is* Way of Being. This is what folks call human. Way of Being defines all you are as human. But not as a *person*. That's up to your absolutely autonomous self, which personally unique, individual Way of Being you develop over time. When you emergently birth during the process of physical conception, your physical body—only two cells in the process of becoming four at this point—builds itself according to the Way of Being that Mina Intentionalized for it that roots in emergent Way of Being.

Way of Being is the nature, or essentiality, of something. It reflects an entity's beingness in the context of *how it is* in relation to the totality of self in the totality of environment. This means the totality of an entity relationally within the totality of not only *its* environment but the local–global environment such as the wholistic natural and supranatural environment and the wholistic universe. For example, people tend to limit the nature of a thing to the thing itself, excluding even its local environment. Sometimes, people include limited aspects of a local environment, such as the lung's nature to expand and contract to move air in and out or to oxygenate blood. But recall that *lung Way of Being* comprehends it wholistically in the context of itself, its anatomical environs, the body as a whole, its physical embodiment, the natural, 'reflective,' and supranatural environments, the universe, All Existence, and ⱭLife's emergent Way of Being.

If one wants to Intentionalize a lung into existence, one needs comprehend its Way of Being and not simply its functional nature, purpose, or essentialities. Doing so is like Intentionalizing a cup of coffee that's not just lacking quiddities like flavor, texture, or aroma, but its wholistic capability to satisfy in every way that one *experiences* it as a person in the world. It's the same with respect to the human body.

Recall our discussion on 'energy' and its pattern in the body. Separate and apart from the energy you think of in ordinary everyday terms, every aspect of your body *is* 'energy.' It isn't merely stuff called matter. It's *matter–Energy*, from archí as the founding 'nodule' of matter–Energy all the way up to your body as a wholistic existent. Each source of 'energy' *is* its own energy pattern. It's unique not just in our universe but All Existence. Your beliefs, mindset, and Thought each has its own energy pattern. What emergent Way of Being Intentionalizes into reality has an energy pattern. What your emergent self Intentionalizes has an energy pattern. These patterns are intrinsic. Each is immutable in and of what it is though mutable when integrating other energy patterns.

Take, for instance, your healthy stomach. It manifests an energy pattern. Then you ingest something that upsets your stomach. It isn't your body's chemistry or a pathogen that upsets it. It's the energy pattern intrinsic of what you ingested clashing—being asynchronous—with the energy pattern of your stomach. The biology, and ultimately chemistry, which medicine ascribes to the upset are only the larger manifestations—symptoms—of this energy pattern clash.

It's the author's repeatable experience that you can entirely remove the effects of the upset by transforming the clashing energy pattern to one that's synchronous, that seamlessly weaves into the fabric of your body. This means *neutralizing* the 'energy.' If you do it quick enough, that's all you need to remove the discomfort. If you wait too long, there's damage inflicted that needs healing and the effect of the 'energy' needs dissipate from that area of your body. When you learn to heal your body, you can do this quickly by Intentionalizing ℒife force in the area to transform the damage. Otherwise, you need await your body's *natural healing* process, which takes longer. 'Natural healing' is what happens when emergent Way of Being ekes past your attributive habits that are Intentionalizing damage into your body. However, if we had 100% mind–brain integration hence 100% awareness thus Intentional power, 'natural healing' would instead be the continually instant manifestation of perfect health regardless damage . . . unless one chooses to Intentionalize imperfect health. We're absolutely autonomous after all.

1.1   Your Body's Dual Way of Being

We've discussed emergent Way of Being in terms of your self-aware proto-energy self. Here, we consider it in the context of your physical body. As a physical, ℒiving entity, your body has its own Way of Being. Since you integrate your body, then emergent Way of Being integrates, too. These two Ways of Being work in tandem in your body. For example, one aspect of your body's ℒiving Way of Being is the natural healing power we observe in every living creature as a function of ℒiving force. However, when emergent Way of Being fully manifests in your body—there are no attributive habits negating it—it augments its limited, ℒiving Way of Being to affect your body's every facet, right down to the DNA and the atoms themselves. This is the root of what people think of as perfect health. In contrast, your body also integrates attributive Way of Being as previously noted and described below. This is the root of what people think of as inevitable illness, disease, and aging.

The reason our world (and each of us) isn't what we all feel deep inside it (and we) could or should be lies in a subconscious response to humanity's addiction to Accountableism's nonautonomous standard of good. It clashed with our emergently autonomous Way of Being at a cellular level so to speak like bad food in our gut grinding at our subconscious on par with a grain of sand in a shoe. This is the real source of our unending sense that we are something more—something better—than how we are today. Individuals imposed Accountableism's Way of Being on their own subconscious 'belief' in larger and larger numbers until it became universal humanity's mindset and every person encountered its 'energy' from the very moment of emergent birth. It wrought a detrimental effect on the spirit-born but absolutely devastated the physical-born with respect to mind–brain integration, physicospirit awareness, and the body's health and wellbeing.

At virtually the same moment in each of our emergent births, we were emergent Way of Being stamped with a nonautonomous, Accountableist, attributive Way of Being. We never noticed the difference except in the deepest recesses of our subconscious that's always encountering thus experiencing the 'energy' of HumanWay of Being, the essence of our self-aware proto-energy beingness.

1.1.1 Attributive Way of Being

Your physical body conceived *as* emergent Way of Being, meaning eternal health and wellbeing. Stamped atop it like a counterfeit image on a coin, however, was your parents' *attributive Way of Being*—even if you popped out of a Petri dish, because, 'energy'—suffused in the nonautonomous Way of Being of Accountableism, which 'energy' *The Story of Life* dubs the Negative Collective Consciousness (neutralized in 2017). The mindset of attributive Way of Being is that you're a physical animal that's a victim of constant biological assault never mind your mysteriously unique mind or spirit or essence. That physical suffering is our natural, even God-given post-Edenic life. That we have to suck it up. Make the best of it. Eat better. Sin less. Hope for redemption or relief. If you don't like it, the solution's obvious: change your subconscious 'belief' from attributive to emergent Way of Being and thereby change your body's physical reality (*Fig. 7.1*).

With attributive Way of Being, damage and defects are inevitable because we subconsciously 'believe' our body is animal. That its only defense against the dark arts of parasites, deadly biological entities, and damage is its own meager immune system augmented with natural medicine or healthier living through chemistry. Emergent Way of Being, on the other hand, arises in Human Way of Being which embodies no concept of damage and defect

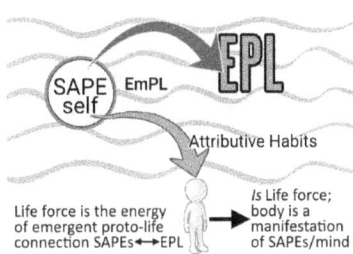

Fig. 7.1. ℒife force is your self-aware proto-energy (SAPE) self plus the 'energy' of the connection twixt SAPE and Energent proto-life (EPL; CH. 2 § 2.3.1:50), which we call emergent proto-life (EmPL). Therefore, your emergent proto-energy self plus EmPL is ℒife force as emergent Way of Being. Your body is a manifestation of mind and is ℒife force, which 'energizes' the matter of your body (CH. 1 pages 2–4).

because it is self-aware proto-energy that is 'energy.' This is ℒife. Your emergent proto-energy, of which you fundamentally are as an emergent being, incorporates emergent Way of Being. It doesn't Intentionalize into your physical body as does attributive Way of Being. It simply *is* your body because its 'energy' *is* the 'energy' of the matter–Energy of every speck and fleck that comprises it. The reason is mind–body integration. Your body went from *unintegrated proto-human*—fertilized egg to two cells going on four—to *integrated human* during the completion of second mitosis. Once integrated, your body *is* the 'energy' of emergent Way of Being, or ℒife force. No other 'energy'—damage, disease, death—can exist in that environment *unless you Intentionalize it*. This is the crux of this book.

When your body integrates subconscious 'belief' and mindset rooted in emergent Way of Being, then what manifests as a result of that integration—note that it doesn't Intentionalize as with attributive Way of Being—is your body *as* 'energy' embodying no concept of damage or defect. It therefore can't manifest damage or defect. It can only do so if that's what subconscious 'wants' it to do, not as a thought process but as an 'energy' reality. Subconscious isn't choosing it like you would a cheeseburger over a taco. It simply exerts its 'energy' reality because your emergent self is an Intentional machine.

This is why your body, in this state of being, can't manifest damage—disease, injury, aging, death—pretty much regardless what befalls it. Emergent Way of Being transforms damage to undamage because nothing can exist in your body that doesn't manifest its energy pattern. Your physical body *is* an energy pattern, not the mere stuff that's matter. As an analogy, think of it in the way that any electromagnetic energy is of a certain pattern. For example, science recognizes gamma rays *as* an overall energy pattern that includes waveform, frequency, modulation, and so on that forms a tangible reality. Similarly, your physical body comprises an overall energy pattern that is uniquely your body. It forms from the energy patterns of individual archí to larger and larger archí substructures, increasing in size to quantum objects and then to molecules, atoms, eventually cells, tissues, and overall shape.

Consider how we can recognize a person from their face, gate, posture, hairstyle, profile, voice, breathing, and many other aspects. If we could perceive energy other than visible light, we would recognize a person by their energy pattern comprising a whole multitude of things like color density, modulation, frequency, waveform, wavelength, and other aspects *in the context of proto-energy* not physical energy like electromagnetism (e.g., infrared, radio). Physical energy is the context people are accustomed to understanding such terms, but we don't describe it in this book.

Your body as an energy pattern cannot be altered without removing some of its energy pattern or injecting a different energy pattern. It's the same with electromagnetic energy of a certain type, say gamma radiation. It can't change without removing energy from, or injecting energy into, the gamma wave that changes its frequency, modulation, and waveform to a different kind of electromagnetic energy. With respect to your body, three kinds of energy can be removed or injected: proto-energy generally, force (e.g., impact or electromagnetic waves), and Intentionalized Thought (from you, another, or Ultraculture). This, of course, is provided your subconscious allows it. Absent your subconscious Intentionally removing your attributive Way of Being such that it no longer negates mind–body integrated emergent Way of Being, it generally does not allow removing energy though generally does allow injecting energy, both on account of subconscious 'belief.' Nothing else changes your body's energy pattern.

Accordingly, if your body fully manifests the energy pattern of emergent Way of Being then no removal nor injection of physical-world energy—say, by a bullet, a virus, a fall, electromagnetic waves—can change that energy pattern. Your state of health is the reality—the 'energy'—of your emergent self, an Intentional machine that *is* the energy pattern of your body. Hence, your state of health can't be changed by anything—any 'energy'—other than your Intentionalized Thought which is subconscious 'belief' and mindset, another person, or Ultraculture and is *of Life* force (the self-aware proto-energy that is you, the person). In this case, your perfect health and wellbeing is immutable absent change by subconscious–conscious attributive Way of Being because mind is omnipotent in the context of your body.

That upset stomach we mentioned earlier couldn't then occur. The instant the 'energy' of what you ingested exerts in your body—a physical manifestation of attributive Way of Being—it immediately synchronizes its energy pattern to the overwhelming 'energy' of emergent Way of Being thus harmonizing with your body's energy pattern. The bottom line here is that awareness of attributive habits generating an attributive Way of Being in your body helps you catch and transform—heal—damage in your body faster and more completely than otherwise.

Section 2
How Your Subconscious Swaps Emergent for Attributive Way of Being

Subconscious 'belief' is 'energy' that is an attributive aspect of your body's Way of Being. We create beliefs about our physical life and body that become subconscious 'belief' thus mindset. It negates emergent Way of Being by subconsciously Intentionalizing attributive habits as an attributive Way of Being which substitutes for emergent Way of Being. As you encounter 'energy' in the world—collective humanity's 'belief' and mindset, ideas, thoughts, physical damage—it pings your self-aware proto-energy self and rings the bell of your mind. This mutates subconscious 'belief' if you allow it . . . well, everyone does because between emergent birth and some level of adulthood, no one knows better and subconsciously habituates it. Subconscious 'belief' then informs mindset.

Accordingly, Mina avers that within about seven days from your third month in the womb—just after self-Intentionalizing your mind—these various 'energies,' which have mutated subconscious 'belief,' diminish emergent Way of Being's influence on your body. Today, on average, emergent Way of Being's influence on your body averages about 0.056% the influence of attributive Way of Being. You can see the reorganization of subconscious 'belief' and mindset happens quickly.

Since your emergent self is an Intentional machine ceaselessly Intentionalizing subconscious 'belief' and mindset into your body—the 'energy' of body *is* the 'energy' of emergent self—you are consistently altering the energy pattern of your body to match the energy pattern of 'belief' and mindset. As this attributive Way of Being energy pattern alters farther and farther from emergent Way of Being's energy pattern, aspects of your body progressively malfunction. An example is the progressive malfunction called aging. It seems to be in accord with your biological environment, but it's really your subconscious influencing your body to manifest malfunction.

When you encounter the 'energy' of a virus or disease or injury that you believe is chronic or incurable, your subconscious experience of this 'energy' (having the 'belief' it's tangibly real and controls your body) Intentionalizes in your body. Your body then manifests these energy patterns into a tangible reality and you find yourself with a cold, virus, cancer, chronic illness or damage, and so forth. In this way, altered subconscious 'belief' and mindset influences the Way of Being of your body until it appears to be naturally susceptible to the world and manifests malfunctions in the same way as an animal body.

SECTION 3
How to Manifest Emergent Way of Being and Avoid Chronic Damage

Quite often in our world doctors will say an injury or illness or their effect is or likely will be permanent, incurable, or worse with time. When doctors tell us this, we tend to believe it almost without a second thought. No doubt, experience seems to prove them right. But are they? Not unless your subconscious 'belief' and mindset dovetail with theirs. Unfortunately, Mina says about 99.991% of humanity's does.

You can change that by developing awareness of your human spirit reality and how your emergent self via subconscious absolutely controls your physical body. Change your subconscious 'belief' about physical human reality where damage is permanent or chronic or inevitable or immutable and you will manifest your body's health and wellbeing. Reversing these effects on your physical body is as simple as becoming aware of your subconscious reality as well as your overall spirit reality. It liberates your subconscious of erroneous 'belief' which, over time—different for each person—allows for more and more aspects of emergent Way of Being to influence a larger and larger percentage (relative to attributive Way of Being) of your Intentional emergent self to bodily manifest health and wellbeing.

Transforming Damage from Your Own Mind

Recall that since your mind is Intentional and brings into reality subconscious 'belief' having the necessary Intentional power—not every belief Intentionalizes—you are the author of most malfunctions in your body except for impact damage not a result of subconscious–conscious choice. This doesn't mean your mind is trying to harm your body. Rather, that in blueprinting its Intentionally powerful 'belief' as your body's attributive Way of Being, your mind—you—alters your body to manifest its reality that age or (chronic) illness, disease, and damage exist therein.

All that's not because such things are, in and of themselves, harmful. They aren't, to humans. It's because your Intentional mind makes them harmful. You remove that reality the same way you created it: Intentionally. In this chapter, we describe that process.

Section 1
Intentionally Heal the Damage

Recall from Chapter 4 § 1 (page 121) that damage is any physical impact or physical change that creates a disruption in the body, that injury as 'energy' trauma is the effect of damage caused by Intentionalized 'energy' from your or another's emergent self, that injury to one's mind is via 'energy' not damage. We've described how to Intentionalize and, here, how to

Intentionally transform your body's health, which you can do or have an Intentional healer do for you (*see* chrismckeon.com/healing-group).

As with a glamour (*see* page 106), damage to your body only exists and continues to exist so long as your subconscious maintains it. The 'energy' of emergent Way of Being exerts *as* the 'energy' of the matter–Energy of your body regardless attributive Way of Being negating its influence. When you let go attributive subconscious 'belief,' emergent Way of Being manifests in your body more and more as 'belief' negates it less and less.

This is similar to the Negative Collective Consciousness (NCC) that dissolved October 13, 2017. Its dissolution meant that humanity's emergent Way of Being of absolute autonomy and mindset without addiction could exert in a felt—experiential—way in each person's mind. Before this, no person in our universe knew they needed to nor even could heal their psyche beyond forgiveness, acceptance, or letting go events. Neither could about 99.99% of people heal their physical body. The 'energy' of the NCC as a universal attributive Way of Being was, until then, too influential.

Despite the NCC dissolving and The Corruption laid bare, damage to the body in the milieu in which we currently live will generally persist for some period of time. This is because it will take several generations for all that 'energy' and erroneous 'belief' and mindset to dissipate individually and collectively. Regardless, emergent Way of Being influencing your body is enough for it to manifest healing in that milieu even without your conscious awareness. Still, in some cases such as late-stage cancer, healing may take longer than your body has time to live according to the damage. So, in the absence of renovating subconscious 'belief' that's manifesting damage in your body, you need employ focused Intentional healing. Until you develop competency in healing—if you even want to—you need a trained healer to effect healing in your body.

1.1 What Is a Trained Healer?

A person who has learned to control their Intentional mind to exert Thought having the Intentional power necessary to effect transformation of the 'energy' of a physical body such that healing occurs is a trained healer. A healer can motivate your subconscious to heal yourself (e.g., Tony on page 204) or else heal your body themselves in spite of your subconscious resistance to healing.

Subconscious resistance arises in a rejection of healing for whatever subconscious–conscious reason a person has. It could be a 'belief' that one deserves pain and suffering, that healing is a sin against God, that material existence precludes it, or a subconscious mindset. These arise in things like guilt, religion, and spiritual or scientific beliefs. Attributive Way of Being is subconscious 'belief' in damage to your body as an inevitable reality of physical existence, whereas subconscious–conscious 'belief' that it's deserved or a sin or against nature roots in Accountableism thus The Corruption. You can subconsciously–consciously accept Accountableism as real—as 'belief'—even having full awareness that your body *is* the 'energy' of emergent Way of Being albeit this inevitably leads to attributive Way of Being. Such subconscious–conscious 'belief' ultimately negates the permanent healing intrinsic of emergent Way of Being.

For example, when a healer heals a person, he or she is Intentionalizing into their physical body their own *L*ife force which is their emergent proto-energy incorporating emergent Way of Being. *L*ife force is the foundational—immutable—'energy' of every person. Beyond emergent Way of Being is individual Way of Being. It is unique in emergent birth. It includes body type such as skin, size, hair, eyes, personality, and beliefs. Unlike emergent Way of Being, it's entirely mutable as an Intentionalized property triggering emergent birth 'in' Energent proto-life. This is the case because the sperm and ovum manifest Intentionalized Thought as physicality as well as 'energy' from biology, parents, ancestors, interfering spirit persons, the NCC (before it dissolved), any local NCC, and The Corruption. In consequence, the fertilized egg manifests all this Intentionality as 'energy.'

When second mitosis triggers emergent birth, it all manifests as an *aspect* of individual Way of Being in the process of emergent birth. The emergently birthed person is, accordingly, emergent *H*uman Way of Being as well as individual Way of Being inclusive of the 'energy' of all this Intentionalized Thought.

A healer does not Intentionalize any change to emergent Way of Being. Rather, he or she Intentionalizes their *L*ife force into the person's physical body that, effectively, is an *attributive* Way of Being that's stronger than the person's *own* attributive Way of Being. Except that a healer's 'attributive Way of Being' is the aforementioned foundational emergent Way of Being, not the 'usual' attributive Way of Being arising in subconscious 'belief' that only manifests harm in the body. This is an analogy, however, not reality.

Anyone can heal themselves or others. *You can heal yourself.* There's nothing stopping you but your own conscious willingness to embark on the journey. Nothing is more exciting and rewarding than discovering the Intentional power of your own mind for yourself. Try it!

Section 2
Damage Can't Exist If You Don't Want It

If you're skeptical your body can heal by the Intentional power of mind then a healer can only heal damage in it temporarily, which means it might return. This isn't *because* you're skeptical or disbelieve. It's because skepticism and disbelief leave subconscious 'belief' unchecked to continue Intentionalizing energy patterns of harm into your body.

For instance, many illnesses or diseases take weeks to years to manifest, as physical-born subconscious Intentionality is so weak. Healed damage would return in weeks to years sooner than originally. A healer would need to heal you again and again. The reason it returns lies in your emergent self (an Intentional, self-actualizing, machine) continually Intentionalizing damaging 'energy' into your body, negating a healer's Intentionality. When you believe you *can* heal but especially subconsciously *want* to heal, the latter lets go its attributive habit Intentionalizing damaging energy patterns into your body. Healing then manifests more than damage like two steps forward one step back instead of the reverse, and the permanence of physical healing improves. Intentional healing is the practice of converting the 'energy' of damage to the 'energy' of emergent Way of Being.

2.1 Permanent Healing

To permanently heal—cure; the effect of healing over time—you need awareness such damage can't exist if emergent Way of Being is the primary influence on how your body functions in the world. A healer can show you how and help neutralize the 'energy' and reorient your subconscious to remove the 'belief' that led to the physical damage you're experiencing.

Healing by a healer is a whole-body experience. It's not a grocery list of items . . . like, if you want to heal your foot, knee, hip, back, neck, a tumor, or anything. Proper healing of the body is wholistic. Healing transforms your whole body, not just a part. However, some things heal sooner than others according to the damage, the strength of the 'energy' involved in the damage, how thoroughly that 'energy' suffuses a particular body part, subconscious 'belief'—attributive habits—Intentionalizing that 'energy,' and how soon you let it go (psyche heal, on the next page).

For example, you may want your prostate or breast cancer healed. You then find other malfunctions healing sooner such as a sore knee, a broken arm, asthma, migraines, and so forth. The stronger your healer, the sooner the damage in your body heals. This is because Intentionality is all about awareness and Intentional power, which is Thought force.

Section 3
Psyche Healing

Although this book is principally about healing your physical body, it's important to introduce you to *psyche healing*. This means transforming from old, harmful beliefs that clear the way for new, unharmful ones that heal your pain and suffering. With psyche healing comes the ability to effect real change in your thoughts, behaviors, and body to undo harmful or self-destructive habits, including physical damage. These pin you like a bug to the board of self-made trials and tribulations.

Psyche healing arises in not merely wanting or wishing for it but desiring it so profoundly, to the very depths of your being, that it rises from thought to Thought to Intentionality. Your conscious desire to let go pain and trauma that you feel in your mind needs reach *critical Intentionality*. This is the moment where subconscious *experiences* conscious Thought and your emergent self thereby Intentionally responds to 'mind energy' with Thought force. It's at this point that psyche healing occurs.

But, it's like peeling an onion. Pain and suffering build up over a lifetime in integrated, referential layers. Psyche healing is letting go layer after layer of built-up pain and suffering integrating you since emergent birth (conception).

Some pain and suffering heals practically instantly and you may feel an instant change in affect. Some heals over minutes, hours, or weeks before you feel some change. Some pain and suffering resists healing because, subconsciously, you don't want to let it go. In this case, you need wait till you're ready or you've Intentionally worked at making yourself ready, or you've healed other underlying pain and suffering first. In the context of what we're teaching here and in *The Story of Life*, psyche healing is only real healing—permanent, as if its pain and suffering never happened—with Mina's involvement. Everything else is merely relief.

Before we get into how psyche healing works, we need discuss the concept of healing, harm, and negative emotive Life force.

3.1 What Is Healing

In the world of traditional healing, there are essentially five types: physical (body), emotional (heart), mental (mind), spiritual (spirit; soul), and holistic (all of these). They're all band-aids on aspects of the self, however. Some don't even exist and anyway heal nothing. For example, it's not possible to heal the physical body of chronic pain or damage without removing proximate negative emotive ℒife force (ℰmℒf; CH. 4 § 1.3.1:123). This section focuses on negative ℰmℒf, but healing necessarily requires neutralizing negative Intentional 'energy,' too, which we cover in Chapter 9.

Unlike physical damage to the body like a cut, impact, or broken bone, the body biologically self-heals over time as emergent Way of Being ekes past attributive Way of Being to manifest healing. A chronic injury is festering 'energy' analogous to gangrene as festering tissue death. Without restoring blood circulation, the chronic malfunction called gangrene inexorably results in the loss of a body part or life. Similarly, without neutralizing negative ℰmℒf, a chronic condition arises that inexorably results in one or more psyche or bodily dysfunctions. In the context of the body, negative ℰmℒf is simply a slow-moving 'gangrenous' condition that humanity has only ever recognized as the inevitabilities of life and especially as aging. But this is mindset, not reality. There are only two modes for healing in our physicospirit context: physical and nonphysical. Underlying both is *harm*.

3.1.1 Healing and Harm

There is no harm in ℒife. It doesn't exist. There's only experience that perceives harm. We tend to think damage or injury constitutes harm (here, damage and injury is synonymous). That's inaccurate because, first, your subconscious–conscious is an aspect of your emergent self-aware protoenergy self and, second, your body has no independent self-awareness. It doesn't *experience* anything. It only *encounters* environment. Thus, neither mind nor body can *experience* damage or injury. You can damage or injure brain but not mind. You can damage or injure the body but it has no self-awareness of it. Your sense that you, the person, *feel* harmed in body or mind is a mindset addiction whereby you *are* body and mind *is* brain, and that these physical components *experience* harm. Yes, one can be shot, stabbed, or physically 'hurt' in some way. But that's *damage*, not *harm* (sol § 1.1.1:362).

Harm is our interpreted experience of physical damage or psychic injury. This is the reason people encounter the same injury yet experience it differently, either as the encountered damage itself or as its experience. Mindset addiction conditions one to view life not through the lens of experience, which one controls, but of encounter, which one doesn't. The more one interprets life through the lens of encounter, the more likely one experiences mind or body harm, which isn't *what* we encounter but *how* we experience it. Only the individual can heal their pain because suffering arises in how one chooses to experience perceived harm's proximate cause or effect. While psyche healing resolves mind pain, it doesn't directly fix damage. Healing resolves harm and then mind–body indirectly heals.

3.1.2 Healing Is Neutralizing Negative Em𝓛F

Every person in our universe experienced the negative EM𝓛F of the Negative Collective Consciousness. This is true regardless one's personal mindset and howsoever one strove to counteract its subliminal effect. Despite its October 13, 2017 dissolution, local NCCs persist until local individuals heal. As an aspect of The Corruption, the NCC was a real force manifesting not just around everyone's mind whereby their emergent 𝓛ife self experienced the 'energy' of its presence, but within the physical bodies of humans and nonhumans. It affected all Living–𝓛ife force beings and 𝕃iving force entities of the natural environment.

Having no awareness of the NCC ourselves, our minds and bodies were nonetheless awash in its negative EM𝓛F. This caused dysfunction quite apart from albeit in conjunction with our own mindsets. Humanity chalked up its physical manifestations to life's apparent aging effect as well as inevitable disease, from the common cold to infectious agents to cancer. Until the NCC dissolved, a person couldn't effectively heal anything because, even if their mindset wasn't conducive to harm and they let go psyche pain to neutralize local negative EM𝓛F and heal their psyche, the NCC's global negative EM𝓛F was ever present. Traditional healers have never known this. Irrespective benevolent intent and healing modalities, they could never *heal* but only *relieve*. Or, failing that, shift the blame by exhorting the healee to be more accountable and to better 'work' the process.

Healing is the practice of neutralizing one's own negative EM𝓛F, including negative Intentional 'energy' as per Chapter 9. When the desire to let go pain is strong enough, one chooses to make it happen. Pain lets go as an aspect of mindset. The subconscious Intentionalizes removing—neutralizing—negative EM𝓛F, excising the Intentionality from one's EM𝓛F that made it a negative 'energy' reality within them, and undoing their choice to experience and embrace their pain. The person thereby experiences a sense of relief, which is a real 'energy' response. It alters mindset and affect, which alters perspective and behavior. Many people experience this aspect of psyche healing every day.

The healing a person needs at any moment is what they're willing to accept, meaning the negative Em𝓛F they're willing to neutralize. Practically speaking this is the pain, suffering, or trauma they're willing to revisit in the context of healing. *Revisit* does not mean to dig up its roots. To work it out. To accept the experience. To integrate it into one's beingness. To use it as a divine lesson or as a way to connect to one's true self or One Source or Higher Power. It simply means having awareness of its reality (not what it is, specifically) and accepting its removal and cessation.

If one has chronic physical or psychic pain, one needs desire healing and then choose it. Energy testing is the modality that opens the way to actual healing instead of the band-aids of traditional healing. Healing the chronic malfunction then happens naturally without further effort on the person's part other than the aforementioned. It takes time according to how much damage the body has encountered (*experience* being interpretive thus subjective, *injury* being damage thus objective), how embodied it is in mindset, and whether one reinstalls—re-Intentionalizes or re-self-actualizes—the same or similar pain.

The bottom line is that healing is Intentionality. One needs bear in mind that wanting, desiring, hoping, and like intentions are *not* Intentionality. Rather, Intentionality is manifesting something as an 'energy'-to-material, external-to-mind reality. In the context of healing, Intentionality means one doesn't *consciously* desire healing; one wholistically, *subconsciously* accepts it—lets go pain and suffering—and chooses it. Your emergent self's Intentionality follows.

3.1.3 Prerequisite to Healing

When individuals can't heal themselves because they're unaware of the possibility or don't know how, yet desire to let go their pain—not simply a conscious want but a subconscious readiness leading to Intentionality—then they need awareness. The person necessarily needs learn the concept of healing—that, indeed, they *can* heal—either through their own process of discovery or by learning it from others. Moreover, one needs recognize they don't necessarily neutralize negative Em𝓛F in its entirety, as they may or may not have let go *all* their pain even though they've chosen to heal.

Healing more often than not involves healing pain layer by layer until fully resolving that aspect of one's pain and suffering. There's a corollary here with the body where resolving one physical pain can unmask a previously undetected pain from damage, chronic 'gangrenous energy,' and so on. Pain layers like an onion because it's referential, an integrated phenomenon that one experiences in consequence of previous pain. For example, experiencing a ruptured relationship as heartbreak means one is prone to experience later events not just similarly but compounded by the previous experience. This is what it means to be 'triggered' by an encounter.

3.1.4 Healing Oneself

When one has awareness they can heal, and knows how or knows a person who knows how, then one is able to heal when recognizing and choosing to let go pain, thus neutralizing its negative EM𝓛F. Presuming that one doesn't re-Intentionalize the same or similar pain in subsequent experiences, *curing* is automatic although the concept of healing pain's many layers still holds as well as mindset addiction's effect on one's sense of harm. When negative EM𝓛F neutralizes, then it's simply *neutral* EM𝓛F—this is proto-love's nominal expression—as an aspect of *collective 𝓛ife force*, i.e., Energent proto-life. Negative EM𝓛F acts as a block to collective 𝓛ife force and, accordingly, a block to proto-love as well. When suffusing a person, negative EM𝓛F essentially deprives one of experiencing universal humanity's collective 𝓛ife force, thus proto-love. Hence, the only proto-love one experiences is what their emergent self exerts in the context of their own counteracting of negative EM𝓛F.

For example, an individual experiences collective 𝓛ife force as his or her neutral, or 'purest,' form of 'energy,' meaning one's unIntentionalized awareness of self and its 'energy' environment. This is one's wholistic state of awareness (SOA) that forms subconscious–conscious mind's SOB–SOA. Negative EM𝓛F, in winnowing collective 𝓛ife force, interferes with this. As a result, humanity's collective 𝓛ife force only partially rises to subconscious–conscious Thought. This is the origin of a person's sense of disconnectedness from life, humanity, or the essence of their own self as a part of greater humanity.

3.2 How Psyche Healing Works

Spiritualists, shamans, doctors, religionists, and more have long practiced healing. However, their methods couldn't *heal* but only *relieve* the psyche. The reason is that actual healing wasn't possible in the context of the Negative Collective Consciousness, and unawareness of reality misdirected their efforts. Pain and suffering root in how one experiences an encounter. Thus, one doesn't heal damage but injury, meaning perception of harm.

The physical body automatically heals so long as negative EmℒF and a mindset unaware of reality aren't restricting ℒife force integrating the body. Unfortunately, pain and suffering ensure negative EmℒF. This restrains our awareness of human reality in The Corruption's milieu despite the Big Healing. It leaves us convinced that life is prone to illness, disease, natural evil, and irremediably short. But that's not human reality (emergent Way of Being). Physicospirit humanity manufactured it in the throes of suffering.

There are two kinds of psyche healing. The first is by the individual, the sort of letting go that many people do at one point or another during their life. The second is real healing that substantively changes the 'energy' of your mind through interacting with Mina, the human person who built our universe and our physical bodies although did not create *you*, the emergently birthed ℘erson. We consider each below.

3.2.1 Healing by Letting Go Pain and Suffering

When a person chooses to let go of pain and suffering, it's a subconscious–conscious event whereby they neutralize—re-Intentionalize—their negative EmℒF. But it's only a partial healing absent Mina, as our universe builder, entangling the person with Energent proto-life (EPL) that 'resets' their ℒife self's awareness of the 'energy' of ℒife force (CH. 8 § 3.2.3:179). Healing is necessarily the individual's choice. Others can only facilitate it or build on it. Since EmℒF is an aspect of ℒife force, it's naturally via ℒife force that one neutralizes its negative expression.

Next, we describe how an individual's psyche heals with Mina entangling him or her with EPL as a full healing modality that renormalizes the individual in terms of the 'energy' of ℒife force (recalling our earlier discussion that humanity lost awareness of that 'energy').

3.2.2 Neutralizing Negative EmℒF

'Negative energy' simply Intentionalizes damage to arise in oneself or another via the individual's attributive habit. Recall that Intentionality is a human-generated fundamental force interacting with Energent–prime and natural as well as supranatural Energent proto-energy. It gives rise to psyche fundamental force that exerts in space as both ideated and emotive Intentionality. Intentionality force is the product of the interaction between Thought force and proto-energy (CH. 6 § 2.1:141).

With matter, for example, fundamental force arises in the interaction between archí force composited from matter–Energy structures and Energent proto-energy. With Thought, on the other hand, psyche fundamental force arises in the interaction between 𝓛ife force composited from a Thought structure and proto-energy of the natural or supranatural Energent. Whether Intentionalizing 'negative energy' in one's mind as negative EM𝓛F—the Intentional interaction between 𝓛ife force and Thought structure—or in one's body as a malfunction or in a way that interacts with other persons or objects, it inflicts harm.

Since pain (and physical disability absent inflicted damage) arises in the context of experience, thus negative EM𝓛F, then its resolution lies in removing it or, more accurately, *neutralizing* it. One accomplishes this with Intentionality as well as by *re*-Intentionalizing one's 𝓛ife force and proto-energy without the Intentionalized damage or with healing Intent.

Mina can't actually psyche heal a person. He can't neutralize your negative EM𝓛F; it's impossible for a person to neutralize another's EM𝓛F. It's a product of, and resides within, your mind despite exerting into the universe such as with the Negative Collective Consciousness. *Pain is your own experience.* No one can change it but the one who chose it—*you*. Simply in choosing to let go, which is an *aspect* of healing, one's subconscious mind naturally exerts Intentional force that neutralizes the particular negative EM𝓛F even if, consciously, the person doesn't know what it is or that they're doing it. Recall that our 𝓛ife self forms an instant state of awareness (SOA) to reality that just as instantly Intentionalizes a particular state of being (SOB) and state of awareness in our conscious mind of Thought which, altogether, is wholistic mind (*SOL* § 1:391). Mina *responds* to subconscious mind's healing as described next.

3.2.3 Healing by Mina

Even though Mina can't neutralize an individual's negative EM𝓛F—an individual does this on their own simply through the act of letting go—he can *fulfill* their healing process. Mina does this by entangling him or her with Energent proto-life. This is what people colloquially think of as God's positive, 'loving energy' enveloping them. A person experiences this in three ways. First, as an influx of 'energy' they experience as *positive*, perceived as loving, emotion. Second, as an awareness that what they're letting go never happened. Third, as a sense of acceptance arising in their partially renewed awareness of the 'energy' of ℌuman Way of Being that Mina Intentionally 'wove' into the 'fabric' of our universe with which they've lost touch—diminished to only a fraction of one's overall awareness—due to The Corruption. We consider each step below.

3.2.3.1 Step 1: Encompassing the Individual with Mina's *Life* force

When an individual genuinely chooses to let go pain, meaning that their subconscious–conscious reconciles to it, one's subconscious immediately exerts that Thought structure as an Intentionality which neutralizes the relevant negative EM*LF*. This is the first aspect of healing. It's not something Mina can force on or induce in a person. Even in personal relationships, Mina as universe builder—for many, a role equivalent to God—is ever unwilling to exert his will upon another unless, on equal footing, he's certain his advice and opinions aren't inadvertently coercing the person. This is an all too common occurrence in people who like, admire, respect, or in some way worship a person whose word, practically speaking, they feel bound to obey. It's a bit like the old American financial services advertisement that, "When E.F. Hutton talks, people listen." This is the reason Mina rejects those aspects of a relationship that elevate him—even in genuine love—where there's any possibility of misconstruing his words or feelings as a divine imperative.

When negative EM*LF* neutralizes, it clears the way for one's *Life* force to 'fill the void.' This is part of healing since *Life* force restores things to their original (peak) condition and nature. It wipes away traumatic 'energy' patterns shackling people to its mental (mindset) and physical (health) rut. It frees them to naturally, successfully change habits, behaviors, and attitudes. While Mina can't heal a person's negative EM*LF*, he neutralizes the 'negative energy' that one's negative EM*LF*-influenced emergent self Intentionalized over time that interacts with mind–body and leads to dysfunction. In the context of 'energy,' recall an individual can Intentionalize literally anything. Although it often results in negative Intentionalized 'energy' in and around others, or a dark cloud following the person that repels others, it most often shows up in the person's own body affecting areas that associate with the 'energy' of the pain they experience.

Once a person chooses to let go pain to heal, this whole train of consequences slows to a halt. The person begins to heal mind then body. When, from time to time, one feels anger, despair, sorrow, hurt, resentment, or any negative EM*LF* rising in oneself, one can refocus Thought and *Life* force to re-Intentionalize—neutralize—it. It then no longer exerts in one's mind although, depending on how long it exerted before they neutralized it, one's mind–body will have already been roiled. One then needs neutralize the effect of that 'energy' in their body and let it dissipate, usually (in our experience) over minutes, hours, or days though sometimes longer (exclusive of damage). One can then choose to focus *Life* force as a healing (restorative) agent. The more one neutralizes negative EM𝓛f and restores affect and bodystate, the quicker and more effective one gets at doing it.

3.2.3.2 Step 2: An Awareness That One's Pain Never Happened

The first person my daughters and I ever healed was *Obāsan*, my children's great-great grandmother from Okinoerabu in the Ryukyu islands of Japan (*TBH/SOL* endnote 54/55). She was filled with anger that her parents had forced her separation from the Chinese father of her baby in Manchuria—Manchukuo, at the time—and sent her home alone. She never again saw her baby while physically alive. American bombs killed her aged 24 at the local airport in the summer of 1945. When her child eventually transitioned to spirit world, she rejected *Obāsan* as her mother.

In spirit world, her family rejected healing when we offered it to *Obāsan* through Mina, scorning and deriding her for even desiring it. As she let go all her pain and suffering and we asked Mina—we called him Creator then—to heal her, my second youngest daughter El could spiritually see the 'energy' and brightness surrounding and suffusing *Obāsan*. This was Mina's 𝓛ife force (before the NCC dissolved, Mina couldn't entangle anyone with Energent proto-life). Her countenance transformed, her energy as a person changed, and happiness and joy exuded from her in such intensity that El was brought to tears and *Obāsan*'s family in spirit world now clamored for their own healing.

When a person simply lets go pain and suffering and thereby neutralizes its negative EM𝓛f harming their psyche, this is the full extent of the healing they get. When one additionally asks Mina to heal them on that basis, their spirit self experiences what *Obāsan* experienced. This change in affect percolates into the person's physically instantiated mind in accord with mind–brain integration . . . for some right away, for others it's varying degrees of later. This is the second aspect of healing.

3.2.3.3 Step 3: Resetting Awareness of the 'Energy' of 𝔥uman Way of Being

When a person emergently births 'in' Energent proto-life, recall it's in accord with 𝔥uman Way of Being of which absolute autonomy is fundamental. The Corruption's intrinsic issue is in leading individuals to reject it for the addictive nonautonomy of Accountableism. This provokes a dichotomy and tension in the psyche between nonautonomy and absolute autonomy because Mina Intentionalized the latter into our universe's very foundation as its warp and woof. Its 'energy' ceaselessly irradiates everything and each one of us.

Universal humanity lost its sensitivity to the 'energy' that *is* absolute autonomy by embracing the nonautonomy of altruistic mindset addiction arising in The Corruption's milieu. Every person lacked awareness, therefore experience, of it. The reason is that the emergent self-aware proto-energy self only has awareness of All Existence beyond—external to—it as 'energy.' This filters into subconscious–conscious mind where the individual experiences it. Without an awareness of this 'energy,' an individual doesn't experience absolute autonomy as it is but only in terms of what it's not, meaning as 'energy' that's not an aspect of Ħuman Way of Being, i.e., the Way of Being which their mind interprets as its own.

If we consider universal humanity absent The Corruption having a 100% baseline awareness of absolute autonomy that Mina irradiates throughout our universe, then our awareness of it in The Corruption's milieu averages only about 0.056%. That's how little the physical-born and spirit-born came to experience autonomy as the Way of Being of Ħuman and of our universe, and why Accountableism became our de facto Way of Being.

The reason for our unawareness was the Negative Collective Consciousness and individual negative EM𝓛F of which, recall, the NCC constituted. The Reconciliation of so-called archangel Michael and Lucifer spontaneously dissipated the NCC. This left universal humanity with only its individual negative EM𝓛F albeit acting as a kind of personal (local) NCC. Accordingly, individual awareness of absolute autonomy's 'energy' remains low despite the Big Healing until individuals progressively neutralize their negative EM𝓛F by letting it go and experiencing the fullness of healing.

As noted, it can be a time-consuming experience to heal pain layer by layer. Mina avers the average individual who's focused on healing can neutralize—resolve—all their layers of pain and suffering in about three years and cure in about another nine years, on average (inclusive of damage). This leaves a person fully healed—not without memories, however—having full awareness of the 'energy' of absolute autonomy irradiating our universe. *Full awareness* means the level of awareness that's humanly capable, not awareness of the full extent of the 'energy' itself.

A person experiences awareness of the 'energy' of absolute autonomy as a direct interaction with the 'energy' of Ħuman Way of Being, which is Energent proto-life. In this way, they subconsciously perceive themselves as transformed and therefore satisfied at such a fundamental, universal level that they can only relate what they're experiencing to being encapsulated in the love of God, Creator, Higher Source, Universal 'energy,' or however they imagine the Ultimate; in a sense, it's orgasmic (SOL CH. 38:595). This is the third and final aspect of healing.

As one progressively heals and awareness of Ꜧuman Way of Being broadens and knowledge of reality improves, he or she never really loses this initial sensorial experience of rediscovering the 'energy' of Ꜧuman. Instead, one relates to it more appropriately the way an adult doesn't throw off childish sensorial experiences in his or her context of limited knowledge even when they've matured to understanding it in light of greater awareness. Here, the analogy means that individuals eventually recognize their birth wasn't evolutionarily random or some (divine) Being's purposed creation. Rather, it's uniquely emergent in accord with pairwise Intentionality in the context of family (SOL § 2:304) since there is no Deific Power, as universe builders are no more and no less ℘ersons like us.

Section 4
Conclusion to Chapters 7 and 8

You are self-aware proto-energy that manifests Thought. What you think is your reality. This is reality inside your mind and, through Intentionality, it is reality in some way, shape, or form outside your mind, too. We emphasize that your physical body is *not* outside your mind. It *is* mind. Its physical matter wholly responds to mind. As you control your subconscious–conscious, so you control your physical body. Whatever you subconsciously want for your body, you get. If you want something different like an end to pain and suffering and excellent, if not perfect, health then you need Intentionalize conscious Thought into your subconscious. Your emergent self will respond. This is psyche and physical body healing.

Your body responds via subconscious to your emergent self. This is because, from the very instant of emergent birth following physical conception, your emergent self then your subconscious integrated—entangled—your body. Emergent Way of Being guided its development along with attributive Ways of Being from your parents, lineage, other people, and all humanity (Ultraculture). You responded to, and then subconsciously-consciously accepted, all this 'energy' into yourself as subconscious 'belief' and, therefore, the Way of Being of your mind and body. To reverse it, you simply remove it from your library of subconscious 'belief' so that Ꜧuman Way of Being predominantly manifests in your mind and emergent Way of Being predominantly manifests in your body.

4.1 My 'Dumpster Fire' Healing

As an example of psyche-cum-physical healing, I experienced a PTSD event in May 2022 I thought I'd healed. It was shattering. Drenched in irrational anxiety and fear. Rooted, Mina said, *in my habituated response* not in the other's action. I focused on changing this subconscious mindset. A week into it I woke up awash in migraines, exhaustion, weakness, heart pressure, and other symptoms like I'd been kicked to death by hoodlums as six decades of 'negative energy' (Em$\mathcal{L}$F) began expelling from my physical body. Spirit persons in the 'reflective' environment (where I argued with the spirit self of the person who kicked this off) saw it as thick, oily, black 'smoke' boiling out of me like a furious dumpster fire, which whiny analogy laying face down on the floor like a corpse got a bark of laughter out of Mina that reflexively popped out of my misery. I'd never experienced anything so painfully devastating. Not even when I broke my spine. I lay prostrate, intense pain within and without, muscles knotted by 40 years of injuries and psyche pain in my back and neck stabbing fire for days.

When my oldest daughter Ayako's spirit self checked in on me, she saw orange 'energy'—Mina entangling me with EPL—around my heart and negative Em$\mathcal{L}$F's black 'energy'—the 'color' as a black-holeness—expelling from my liver. Mina said it would last a week and it did. The agony released and dissipated over several more days. My body *felt* healed—muscle knots, internal symptoms gone though headaches for several days more—even if bone-wearily, stagger-mode haggard. My biological energy had significantly upgraded, which shut down all but sway testing, and altogether necessitated a two and a half month recovery. My psyche felt restored to the unwoundedness of childhood. Relaxed. Untroubled. *Healed*.

My unusual healing was predicated on nearly five years with Mina. It's not an example of what you need or will experience since suffering is unique. It just conveys the physical effect on the body of healing one's mind.

Next, we describe transforming damage to your body from others' Intentionality.

Transforming Damage from Others' Intentionality

Mind is Intentional. It brings your subconscious–conscious Thought or subconscious 'belief' having the necessary Intentional power into physical reality (remember, not every thought or belief necessarily Intentionalizes). This is true for every person. Thus, anyone in the universe can cause or coax a malfunction in your body however random or traceably caused by some incident it appears to be.

Mina reports that about 27.5% of all physically alive persons on Earth experience only one maliciously damaging Intentional attack on their bodies and about 44% two or more. Additionally, for about 24% of all physically alive persons, Intentionality damaging the body is unintended, meaning accidental. Altogether this adds up to about 90% of all physically alive persons experiencing Intentional damage to their bodies. It's not all doom and gloom. About 98.3% of the physically alive experience Intentional healing, mainly from spirit persons but the physically alive as well. You may think your body is a self-existing entity distinct from all but physical forces, but it exists primarily in the human (thus, Intentional) environment not the physical one.

Bear in mind that, from Mina's perspective, Intentional healing absent permission is an attack on the body as much as Intentional malice despite the one undoing damage while the other creates it. The reason is that, without permission, Intentionalizing an effect into someone's body denies their autonomy, the fundament of Ꜧuman Way of Being. Think of it like force feeding someone who isn't hungry or dislikes the menu or, as Mary Baker Eddy noted, "to enter a house . . . displace the furniture, and suit one's self in the . . . management of another man's property" (*Misc. Writings,* 283:4). Therefore, never heal without permission.

People use two means to Intentionally attack—damage—a body: direct and indirect Intentionality. *Direct* Intentional attack—exerted 'energy'—is when a spirit person or a physically alive person (or their spirit self) Intentionalizes 'energy' directly in or around your body or body part to cause damage (*Fig. 9.1*). Here's how it works. The person manifests their Intentional Thought in the desired spatial location of your 'reflective' body or body part to effect a force or the 'energy' of damage. Recall your 'reflective' body is the 'mirror' of your physical body in the 'reflective' environment.

Whatever force your 'reflective' body encounters in the 'reflective' environment—a shove, say—only about 10% of that force translates to your physical body. For example, a spirit person whacks a baseball bat across your 'reflective' knee or body slams your 'reflective' body like a linebacker where, in the natural environment (the physical world), your knee would snap or you'd be pâté on the ground. However, only about 10% of that force translates from your 'reflective' body to your physical body owing to the difference between the natural and supranatural Energents. You might physically feel a sharp pain, a jolt, an unexplained surge in motion, or a momentary loss of balance.

An Intentional attack in the 'reflective' to give you some knee pain could be Intentionalized 'energy' of damage *within* the 'reflective' knee. Your physical knee would feel about 10% of that 'energy' as pain. Your own subconscious, having a 'belief'—attributive habit—that the pain is real, would then Intentionally exert that 'energy' of damage, which mind–body integration then manifests as a physical reality.

Despite what others are Intentionally doing, it's only ever your mind— *you*—that makes your body manifest illness, disease, chronic damage, and all the rest. This is because no person can *directly* but only *indirectly* manifest damage in your body.

Indirect Intentional attack affects your body when your subconscious thus emergent self Intentionally responds to it. This means your subconscious experiences another's Intentionalized 'energy,' which is to say, your emergent self exerts the latter's 'energy' into your body as a reaction. Figure *Fig. 9.1* shows another person Intentionalizing knee pain in or around your

Introduction to Transforming Damage from Others

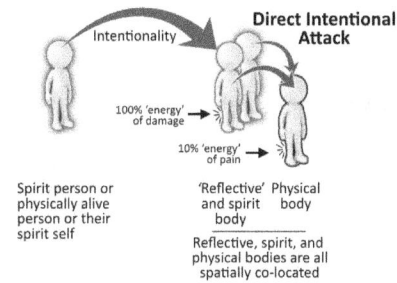

Fig. 9.1. Example of direct Intentional attack. A spirit or physical person (or their spirit self) Intentionalizes hostile or malicious 'energy' of damage into your 'reflective' knee. About 10% translates to your physical body and you experience pain. Your embodiments are spatially co-located. Thus, the Intentionalized 'energy' pings your subconscious, which Intentionally reacts according to 'belief.' Mind–body integration means it manifests in your body since body is subconscious.

knee. Your subconscious perceives the 'energy' because your spirit self is spatially located with your 'reflective' body thus your physical body. If we were to spatially locate the 'energy,' it would be one foot or less from or even within your 'reflective' body. If it pings your subconscious—rings the bell of your mind—then it *experiences* this 'energy' *as* knee pain.

Based on its attributive habit—'belief'—and regardless how 'energy' arrives on your subconscious doorstep, it reacts *as* 'energy.' That is, like gasoline-soaked tinder explodes in flame at the tiniest spark, your emergent self detonates Intentional 'energy' at the mere whiff of Intentionalized Thought. The reaction is driven by your attributive habit. Maybe your mindset is that your knee is strong, without previous injury. In this case, emergent self detonation may only generate a twinge or an ache. If you've fretted over the years of re-injuring your knee, then your emergent self's reaction is a powerful surge of Intentional 'energy' into your knee that makes your eyes water. This is as true for the 'energy' of a cold, flu, or maybe a swollen prostate in your sixties or the breast cancer your mother had as it is for your subconscious–conscious awareness that the effects of aging increase year over year.

So, your emergent self reacted. Symptoms of a new or old knee injury show up. You feel pain and debility. This is not the attacking person *directly* inflicting knee pain on you. Instead, it's you *indirectly* exerting their Intentional Thought as your own Intentional 'energy' into your knee by means of Intentionally powerful subconscious 'belief' or conscious belief. This happens because your subconscious is habituated to respond to such 'energy' as real damage to your body, as if you had just physically smacked your knee on a low table. The pain *is* your attributive habit. The debility—damage—that follows *is* attributive habit. It isn't a *part* of your body. Your subconscious 'belief' manifests it *as* your body.

It's only physical damage if *you* subconsciously make it so. Your subconscious could reject another person's Intentional 'energy.' In this case, although your subconscious perceives the 'energy,' it need not react to—experience—it. Its bell isn't rung because there's no attributive habit provoking a reaction. Even if you did bang your knee on a low table, the 'energy' of damage that your subconscious perceives in the objectively physical blow couldn't manifest in the knee's environment where the 'energy' of emergent Way of Being is manifest.

With an attributive habit, the 'energy' of damage might be your emergent self manifesting through Intentional mind–body integration the 'energy' of bruising, kneecap damage, swelling, and so on. Furthermore, the damage could persist as chronic and progressively debilitating depending on the attributive habit. Having no such habit in this scenario means none of that happens. Your knee feels and operates fine regardless how hard you smacked it. That's your subconscious unfettered by attributive Way of Being.

So, yes, another person can Intentionalize 'energy' harmful to your body. But if your subconscious rejects it—does not Intentionally respond to it—then it's without effect. The ultimate source of Intentionalized 'energy'—from you or other persons—is immaterial to your subconscious. The 'energy' your self-aware proto-energy self encounters and your subconscious experiences, to which your emergent self Intentionally responds, affects your body's Way of Being, your subconscious 'belief,' and mindset. In the above example, it reinforces your *L*ife mind's attributive Way of Being as well as that of your body.

Accordingly, no person can Intentionalize harm into your body. They can only Intentionalize the 'energy' of harm that your self-aware proto-energy self encounters and your subconscious experiences. If emergent Way of Being fully manifests in your body then the 'energy' of damage can't affect your body because your emergent self won't Intentionalize any 'energy' that's inconsistent with emergent Way of Being. If, on the other hand, your attributive Way of Being (which negates emergent Way of Being) manifests in your subconscious, then it's your own emergent self Intentionalizing another's Intentionalized 'energy' of damage into your body, which reinforces your body's attributive Way of Being. This manifests physical damage in your body as a malfunction that people feel as injury, illness, disease, chronic damage, and so on.

The critical takeaway here is that you are not a victim of human and other 'energies' of our universe in which your physical body is awash. Because you're an Intentional being having full control of your body, you are never a victim. Your mind is omniexistent. Omnipresent. Omniscient of itself. Omnipotent in the context of embodiment. It outweighs all else through Intentionality. Only to the extent that your subconscious Intentionalizes into your body the harmful 'energies' it experiences (from whatever source) are you a victim . . . of your own subconscious.

Whatever happens to you, in some way you subconsciously–consciously chose to *experience* it the way you did, even if you didn't choose to *encounter* it. This means you need gain awareness and control of your subconscious to experience a physical life of perfect health. You remove the imperfect health originating in another person's Intentionality the same way that *you* subconsciously created it: Intentionally. In this chapter, we describe that process.

Section 1
Awareness of an Attack

Presently, no person on Earth manifests emergent Way of Being as their body's Way of Being. People instead manifest attributive Way of Being to greater or lesser degrees vis-à-vis emergent Way of Being. For some, emergent Way of Being more prevalently manifests versus attributive Way of Being Intentionalizing. Their bodies thusly experience better health. For others, it's the reverse with worse health.

On average, people presently experience a physical health that reflects emergent Way of Being influencing their body only about 0.056% compared to attributive Way of Being's influence of about 99.944%. Therefore, everyone to a greater or lesser degree suffers from their own Intentionalized malfunctions in their body. These originate either in their own subconscious 'belief' directly, or in the subconscious 'belief' or conscious belief of another person indirectly. Regardless origin, you and you alone attack your body's health and wellbeing through your own 'belief' and mindset.

1.1   Intentional Attack

Another person attacks you when, perhaps wanting to punch you in the mouth or employ some cancel culture against you, instead settles for consciously (and Intentionally) wishing you harm or else subconsciously exerting some specific 'energy' of damage. These attacks work because, fundamentally, one's subconscious mind believes their body is vulnerable to nature. When one encounters and experiences the 'energy' of such a vulnerability then he or she literally manifests it via Intentionality *as* their body's reality (no different from a malicious person stoking one's pet fear to elicit a desired response). This is the origin of why some folks are sickly and others never sick, why some die of non-fatal damage and others survive what any doctor calls fatal. It isn't magic. Genetics. Luck. God. It's *your* Intentionality. *Your* doing. *Your* will.

This doesn't mean that other people, including spirit people, can't help you. They do. Spirit persons who care about you Intentionally mitigate damage to your body; it's helpful if you're not subconsciously negating it. Or they use Intentional energy to affect problematic physical forces. The attempted assassination of Donald Trump on July 13, 2024 is a case in point. Here, certain spirit persons used Intentionality to physically alter the trajectory of the bullets as well as to provoke Trump to move his body, not head, off the crosshairs. We live in a world filled with spirit humanity as much as we do with physical humanity, and many of them are not idle.

It's our lack of awareness of how we exist in the world that seemingly makes us vulnerable to nature through our or another's Intentional attack. And that's what it is: an attack. You attack your body the same way you attack yourself with self-recrimination, guilt, self-hatred, or self-harm. Quite often, self-hatred or depression manifests in the body as a malfunction. This is why psyche healing is important to healing your body; you can't heal a malfunction that your self-hatred or guilt or depression is every day in every way replenishing like a zombie virus.

Another person consciously, or more usually subconsciously, attacks your body with much the same Thought that you, in the same way, consciously or subconsciously attack yourself. Their attack (of which you're unaware) is analogous to you hating on yourself and then another person chiming in to agree. In such a recriminative state of mind, this only leads you to double down on yourself. An attack subconsciously rings the bell of your mind. That 'note' resonates and Intentionally affects your body.

Section 2
Neutralize an Attack's Energy

Do it yourself or ask a healer. This entails using Intentionality to strip the 'energy' of its Intentional effect, effectively neutralizing it. Recall that proto-energy suffuses our universe and, accordingly, our bodies. The unique power of the human mind is its ability to exert Thought in such a way that proto-energy responds to it. It thus takes on Thought's characteristics similar to the way that air, in the form of a sound wave, takes on the characteristics of one hand clapping the other. As with Intentionality, the energy of sound is quite capable of harming your body, so Intentionality isn't as alien as it may first appear.

Neutralizing the 'energy' of an attack simply re-Intentionalizes proto-energy's 'neutral' interaction with your body until your own Thought re-Intentionalizes it either with your erroneous subconscious 'belief' about your body's vulnerability to nature or your 'belief' that the 'energy' of the matter–Energy of your body *is* the 'energy' of emergent Way of Being. This is how an injury that's healing may suddenly and inexplicably turn for the worse or else unexpectedly heal as if by magic.

Although proto-energy's interaction with our bodies is 'neutral' as a baseline, the reality is that we live in a human milieu, a veritable forest of Intentionality. Living in it is no different than living in air that's pristine or polluted. You protect yourself from the latter with a respirator, filter, or mask. Similarly, you protect yourself from harmful Intentionality with a 'belief' and mindset that neutralize it. The latter roots in emergent Way of Being that physical health arises in mind not body. That body can't be harmed. That ℒife doesn't depend on nature. That you have ℒife suffusing your body, which consequently has all of ℒife's characteristics. You heal the damage of harmful Intentionality originating external to own-self in the same way you heal damage from your own mind, which we describe in Chapter 8 § 1.

Section 3
Conclusion to Chapters 1–9

You are not your body. The science conceit that what's observable (at least, observably comprehensible) is all that's real, that if it can't be observed then it doesn't exist, is a plank in the eye. Its belief that the lack of evidence for anything spiritual not directly observable constitutes evidence for its nonexistence has bamboozled humanity into believing we're nothing more than a smarter monkey with an ineffable mind rooted only temporally in the neuronal discharges of our evolutionarily sophisticated brain.

Science likes to figure it's mathematically probable that a monkey can produce Shakespeare (presumably the Bible, too, if not *Catch 22*) with enough time and random clacks. But this begs a strictly materialistic reality that discounts everything that makes humanity human. And it's entirely false. It ignores every other aspect of our human self that's ever trying to push its way out of the shadows of myopic scientific reasoning. People intuitively know this even when they rationally reject it. Science uses intuition as a tool to reach new understandings so long as it can reason it out around observational experience.

But science wholly ignores intuition when it doesn't seem to fit the jigsaw puzzle that it thinks it's assembling. Not only the hard sciences but soft sciences like psychology certainly give nods to the power of mind or subconscious. Yet, they rein in hard when that inevitably leads one to postulate much less experience spontaneous healing.

3.1 Energy Testing

If you want to heal what medicine can't or is anyway unaffordable then it's necessary to expand your definition of the principles of the scientific method and human reality. The beauty of energy testing (ET) is that, like any scientific experiment to test a hypothesis or predict an outcome, ET answers can be energy tested across a diverse group. Aggregated ET responses necessarily lead to the same conclusion that scientists arrive at (and is the best they can expect): that something, in this case Intentionality and Intentional healing, is more or less likely accurate with respect to physical reality. And one can empirically test it as well.

We reference energy testing as data that one objectively formulates as information, knowledge, and wisdom similar to that acquired via the scientific method. As you acquire experience, develop your ET competence, proficiency, and skill and establish your own reliability baselines, you can verify what you read in this book. To the extent you connect with a local or global ET community, you can test your understanding and interpretation of it individually and in the context of others (*see* toteppitpress.com/et-community).

Quite simply, ET is chakra energy interacting with the body's biological energy. Even if you have neither knowledge nor conscious awareness of ET, your physical body always responds to chakra energy. If your chakras are sufficiently 'open' with awareness (CH. 9 § 3.1.2:193; *SOL* § 1.2:634, § 2.3.4:526), chakra energy sways your body to a greater or lesser degree.

3.1.1 What Is Chakra Energy

Chakras only have meaning in the context of the natural environment. They aren't magical portals to spiritual enlightenment, oneness with the

Eternal, or perfect health. It's more productive to think of chakras in toto as a specialized organ no different from, and just as necessary as, any other organ and having a twofold purpose. First, they integrate the body with the natural environment in a way the physical senses rooted in neural impulses can't. Second, they integrate ℒife—the self integrating the body—with the natural environment inclusive of the 'reflective' environment wherein a physicospirit person can interact via ET or their spirit self with the spirit selves of other physically alive persons as well as with spirit persons visiting from, or presently in, spirit world.

The 'energy' of your chakras is biological 'energy' arising in 𝕃iving force interacting with matter–Energy as described. It's similar to the way real energy (fundamental force) arises in the interaction of proto-energy with matter–Energy. In a sense, chakra energy is the 'fundamental force' of the 𝕃iving body just as actual fundamental force is of the universe.

Chakra 'fundamental force' constitutes the chakra version of applied energy E, which determines the behavior of our body vis-à-vis everything in the 'reflective' environment inclusive of spirit persons. It also exerts the 'energy' of what the physically embodied person thinks–feels and awareness–experiences (*enimerótis–empeiría*; see SIDE NOTE on page 146) as a physicospirit person. This 'energy' is 'visible' in the sense it is felt–perceived by spirit persons in the 'reflective' environment as well as by any physical entity 'reflected' therein from microbe to monkey; they feel–perceive the physically alive's chakra energy as it interacts with the 'reflective' environment's proto-energy (its 𝕃iving force). Thereby, they feel–perceive the physicospirit person's SOB–SOA (state(s) of: being, awareness) representing thoughts and feelings—essentially, how energy testing works (SOL § 2:625)—and nonhuman physical entities can feel–perceive aspects of bodystate–mindstate in accord with their capacity.

3.1.2 Chakra Health

You have seven chakras: crown, pons, lung (traditionally, throat), heart, solar plexus, lumbar (sacral), and root. All chakras need be sufficiently 'open' for accurate, reliable ET. Even if only one of the seven is 'closed,' that is sufficient to render your ET inaccurate.

A 'closed' chakra means it is minimally interacting with 𝕃iving force via the aura. This reduces overall chakra energy movement in your 'reflective' body, thus your physical body's biological 'energy' interaction with the full picture. One or more 'closed' chakras are analogous to vapor lock reducing fuel flow to an engine. Nevertheless, chakras never truly 'close,' they simply integrate Intentionalized Living force *as* chakra energy at a 10% minimus. But this is a functionally 'closed' state for energy testing. Over time, 'closed' chakras result in your biological 'energy' having insufficient sensitivity to chakra energy. As they 'open' more for longer, your biological 'energy' sensitivity to chakra energy naturally improves. When you develop awareness of this phenomenon, you can consciously utilize it by focusing on—having awareness–experience of—a specific 'frequency'–resonance (SOL § 1.2.1.2.1:499).

'Frequency'–resonance arises in your physically-instantiated mind's state of being (SOB) and state of awareness (SOA), and that of spirit persons in the 'reflective' or supranatural environment who focus on a physical person's *focal mindstate* (Thought; SOL § 4.1.1:378). In this way, you can interpret your body's 'frequency'–resonance response to chakra energy in the context of focal mindstate, meaning a *query*—a question or affirmative statement posed, or conscious thinking–feeling—to which a spirit person responds. When you query a spirit person, they choose to respond to you. As their response interacts with your aura in the context of the 'reflective' environment, it gives rise to chakra energy in your 'reflective' body having a specific 'frequency'–resonance consistent with your query. You interpret this via your awareness–experience of it as (sway test) 'movement' in your body. This is basic energy testing.

3.1.3 The Aura

What the ancient and modern traditions call minor chakras or 'energy' centers aren't chakras at all in the sense of 'energy' vortices or toroidal flow structures, but locally 'frequency'–resonance areas of the aura. All human and nonhuman physical bodies have an aura. It arises in the physical body's matter–Energy interaction with Living force as a real energy Υ entity that encapsulates the 'reflective' body in the 'reflective' environment.

Read Chapter 29 in *The Story of Life* for all you need to know about your chakras and aura. For the final chapter of this book, we turn to testimonies written by five individuals Intentionally healed by the author.

Testimonies

This chapter provides six Intentional healing testimonies by persons the author healed with Intentionality. Each wrote their experience and approved the publisher's edits for style, grammar, and readability. Real names are used with permission unless '(P)' follows. An envelope image next to a name indicates he or she is willing to accept correspondence regarding his or her testimony. Provide the publisher the name(s) of whom you'd like to contact at toteppitpress.com/contact. He or she may respond to you directly or via the publisher.

Simon ✉

I am 70 years old and married 42 years and happily raised three daughters and two sons. The first sign that something was medically amiss goes back five or six years. At times, I experienced tunnel vision followed by a sensation of blacking out. I never lost consciousness, but the episodes grew more frequent.

My doctor shocked me with my blood test. It showed I had become a Type 1 and Type 2 diabetic. He called mine "runaway" diabetes. My glucose levels were off the charts. If untreated, he said that blindness, loss of limbs, stroke, heart attack, even death were all too common. Worse, I had also developed erectile dysfunction (ED). If nothing else, this got my full attention! On top of it all, I'd been dealing with hypertension (high blood pressure) for more than 25 years which I controlled with medication.

My diabetes prognosis pushed me down hard. My doctor and all the literature said it was a lifelong condition. Incurable. I couldn't accept this easily and argued with my doctor.

"Wouldn't it be more prudent if doctors just admitted that, at this time, the medical profession just doesn't *know* how to heal its cause? That—"

"No, no, no . . ." He wasn't taking my remark with very much humor.

"—therefore, you're only treating the symptoms? Not dealing with—"

"Simon, that's the stages of grief talking. Just take your medications as I've prescribed them. You'll be fine. It is what it is."

Well, being German, following orders is no big deal. The doctor knows best. I've believed in the power of medicine all my life. After looking into it, I found that a change of lifestyle contributes to ameliorating this condition. But diabetes needs constant attention *and* medication to keep it under control. I had no choice but to go along with the program, as Americans like to say.

"Take meds," they said. "Lose weight. Exercise. Eat 'healthy' foods."

"Bah!" I grew up with potatoes, bread, pasta, sausages, cheese, and meats of all sorts. I was not a happy camper. Instead of obeying the healthy diet rules, I'd rather take more of the medication and maintain a happy lifestyle than a 'healthy' one. My doctor prescribed three different types of medication to control my diabetes. To add insult to injury, the co-pay for a 90-day supply of one of them was about $650! *Made in Germany*. I had to laugh. This sums up where I was, health-wise, in September 2023.

A friend told me about *The Story of Life* book by Christopher McKeon and gave an 'elevator' explanation about it over the phone. Since the online version is free, I tried it only to learn that I am too old school for eBooks. I needed a 'real' copy. A printed book. The book's subtitle is: *A Shocking Revelation About God and the Universe to End Fear and Liberate Humanity*. And for sure it shocked me. It still *is* shocking me!

Ultimately, I found the book leads to healing. Not just physical healing, which was very important to me. After all, our human body is a 'biological machine' albeit, I admit, a sophisticated one. But just as important to me, the book leads to psyche healing. I am not only my physical body. Most essentially, what makes me human lives in my mind, not in my organs.

I read through *The Story of Life* but English is not my first language. I thought that I had a pretty good command of the language only to find out it is, in reality, somewhat below average. Facing this challenge, I committed to look up every word I didn't understand because making assumptions can and will lead to misunderstandings. I didn't want that when learning about healing myself. If this is for real, I thought, then I had better dig into it well. And I am extremely glad I did.

In the summer of 2023 and 2024, the author held a seminar to discuss *The Story of Life*. He was open to answering any questions my friend and I might have. I attended with gusto. This is when the subject of healing came about, and he addressed it thoroughly.

I learned that one of *The Story of Life*'s main goals is healing. Not just the body, but almost first and foremost our psyche. My little testimony here does not have the space or purpose to explain all the 'mechanics' of healing. I simply wish to let you know the result which I experienced. I highly recommend reading for yourself what leads to healing and how.

Christopher added me to his healing group. There is no charge for it at the time I am writing this testimony. So, that was a big plus when diving into something new and unknown. Also, Christopher is in Colorado and I live in California. But I learned that distance doesn't matter to the healing that he does. After about three months being in his healing group, I experienced hypoglycemia on several occasions. This refers to dangerously low levels of glucose in the blood. My symptoms were shaking, inability to stay focused, and bordering on confusion. I was taking my daily medications and was careful to keep a close check on my glucose levels. At times it was below 50 mg/dL.

I called my doctor. He said, "Stop all your diabetes medications at once! And get your blood re-evaluated."

I couldn't believe it. But the results surprised—I might say, shocked—us both. He advised me to stay off the medication and keep an even closer watch on my glucose levels. Well, after about four months and without any diabetes medications at all, my glucose levels have stayed in the 'acceptable' range. What I mean is that, if I indulge too liberally as far as food is concerned, my glucose levels spike. But then they recede toward normal rather quickly as if I didn't have diabetes.

One aspect is important to me, and surely for others who have diabetes. While taking my medications, it was nearly impossible to skip a meal without experiencing symptoms of hypoglycemia. After my healing in the healing group, I can now miss meals as often as I want without feeling any signs of hypoglycemia. None.

What I appreciate from Christopher's book, his seminars, and his healing activities is that there is more to it than simply accepting healing. It involves me, my own self, in ways that pushes into realms that make us truly human. This includes my subconscious mind and beyond. I had to ask myself: am I truly willing to let go of my pain and suffering to heal? It seems a silly question on the surface, but is it truly? Once again, I found out the hard way that it may not be as easy as it sounds. Especially when I discovered through Christopher's energy testing that my conditions have been almost entirely self-inflicted. And this is where the real effort begins: healing my psyche. I wouldn't call it work, exactly. Just a desire and an effort to have conscious awareness that I want to heal. Then the body will naturally heal with it. And that was my experience.

Let's talk about ED. It's not an easy topic for many men to discuss, because it feels like it diminishes one's 'manhood.' To my way of thinking, the ability to have a warm, intimate, close, caring, and loving conjugal relationship with my spouse has been the gasoline that powers my engine. To limit this to a 'spiritual' relationship, or else to focus only on our 'emotional' connection does not cut it for me. Who enjoys a good soup without salt? It was and is a pivotal aspect to my life that keeps our healthy relationship going.

During my ED challenges, I noticed I had become too intimidated by it to approach my wife. Fear of failure only exacerbated it. A vicious cycle began. The pharmacy has a 'solution' for it in various pills and potions, but these gave me negative side effects. When my healing began through Christopher, can you imagine the joy and happiness I felt when my ED went down and my performance went up (no pun intended)? It is still healing as of the time I am writing this testimony because it has lasted now for years. But, besides clearing up subconscious issues that I am currently still working on, it *is* healing. And I couldn't be happier.

The third medical issue I want to mention is hypertension, or high blood pressure. It has been a part of my life for over 30 years. I began taking medication for it 25 years ago. As of this writing, it has not yet fully healed. But it *has* healed. I am confident it will fully heal.

Just as I check my diabetic blood, I measure my blood pressure daily. Prior to when Christopher began my healing, my hypertension was not well controlled even with my all my medications. It has always been around 145/100/95. This is the systolic/diastolic/heart rate, and these numbers are considered too high. Whenever I forgot to take my pills, my blood pressure shot up to around 200/120/95. Now, after healing for 3-5 months, it is consistently around 120/80/80 with my medication. And sometimes it even falls below 120. I watch the numbers carefully.

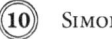

Consulting with my doctor and checking my daily numbers, I feel confident that the prescribed dosage will go down as my healing continues. Ultimately, my goal is no more drugs for this condition.

Finally, what about psyche healing? It turns out that letting go of pain and suffering is not as easy as it sounds. Since we are all unique, for which I learned to thank God over nearly a lifetime in my church, there must be infinite shades of grey to what I am trying to explain.

During my life, I came across several people who, consciously or subconsciously, knew how to make me miserable. Some of them had a certain amount of authority over me. Every time these names or memories popped into my head, I had 'trigger' moments: a sensation of utter frustration, anger, bitterness (not hate, but close to it), and helplessness. To this day, I have traumatic dreams where I find myself 'trapped,' replaying the circumstances surrounding these memories. I despise these dreams—well, nightmares—and wish for them to just go away.

After reading *The Story of Life* many times and attending two healing seminars, I have come to understand that I actually had a choice. But at the time, my mindset limited my perceived options as to how I could, or was allowed to, respond. Looking back, I find myself dealing with feelings of guilt and regret at being a coward for not standing up to these bullies. All these detrimental experiences screwed themselves into my mind like a long bolt of pain. If you wish, you can replace the word 'screwed' with 'F-ed.' That's certainly how it felt—like stories of prison rape. What is weird is that I learned how it was *me* who 'allowed' these conditions to bore into my mind.

Regardless whether one is atheist, agnostic, or zealously religious, these emotional sensations are not mentally healthy. They are called negative emotive life forces for a reason. Over time, they became destructive in me, making me mentally and physically sick. Yet, I persisted in practically hating these people who victimized me. Something like a guilty pleasure, I suppose. I liked to indulge in my negative feelings. They sort of pumped me up. Or riled me up. It was almost like I enjoyed my negativity. Until I read *The Story of Life* and talked to Christopher at the seminars and then over many, many phone calls.

You see, unbeknownst to many, including myself, these negative feelings are not only destructive to me but to the other person (the victimizer), too. I discovered they'd boomeranged on me, making me even more mentally and physically unhealthy. My negative, vengeful feelings were sort of like a curse I had directed at them but unknowingly onto me, as well. When I understood this, I realized it was just another vicious cycle. Since it was self-destructive, I had to let go. I hope this describes to some extent why one wouldn't want to let go of their pain and suffering so easily, and why it is not such a silly question after all.

All I can say is that to the extent I truly longed for, wished for, and hoped for healing, there is also a need in me to let go. Let go of what? My understanding of that is part of my homework, to figure out what it is that I need to let go. But now I can always ask for help, can't I? I am now in a much better place mentally and physically.

Shelley (P)

My story begins in New Braunfels, Texas in September, 2023. I was becoming anxious as I was looking at having to surrender my car to the bank because of financial hardship. I gave up the car in October. I felt depressed. Trapped. I had never been without a car. I felt that I had lost my freedom.

My health was declining with all my stress. In December I went to the dentist for a cleaning. They told me my blood pressure was high and they couldn't continue. I rescheduled. I was frightened by the bad news piling up and, unawares, was manifesting shortness of breath and dizziness and heart palpitations quite often, which required that I lay down to rest.

Then I called a friend, who is a Christian Science practitioner [healer], for help through prayer. I have relied on Christian Science for healing all my life and she has helped me over many years whenever I didn't feel well. This time, she told me there was a new way that I could look at my life and wellbeing. She said it would really help me feel more confident with a more enlightened, a more aware, understanding of how my body and mind worked. She had taken what she knew about mind through her study of Christian Science and translated it into a more complete picture. This came from her new understanding through *The Story of Life*, published in 2022. She discussed some parts of the book with me and introduced me to a new concept of God that I found even more useful than what I'd always had. Well, at my next dental appointment my blood pressure was still high, but not so high that I couldn't make it through the cleaning.

The book explains that a human being named Mina actually built our universe and is the Intentional mind that determined how it works. He built our universe to make sure we had total autonomy. This is the true, natural way of being for every human. This means that we are never judged or punished by him regardless the actions we choose. We're able to live free of guilt and self-condemnation. He never initiates rules for us to live by or determines our state of health and well being. He built this universe to give us the best eternal life possible. Therefore, we are not under the rules of a judgmental God who determines whether we go to heaven or hell because of the choices we made in the circumstances of life in which we found ourselves. This was very liberating for me.

As time moved on, I continued feeling short of breath and dizzy at times. That was very scary. A relative asked me if I wanted to go to the local clinic for a check-up. I agreed to go. They checked my blood pressure and it was too high. The doctor prescribed the least amount of blood pressure medicine he could in recognition of my Christian Science faith and advised me to see a family physician at a later time. I took the medication for a few days, but began feeling bad again. My blood pressure on the medication was now too low. I called my friend. We agreed that I would stop taking the pills and rely for my treatment and healing on the new understanding she was teaching me. That was a relief. No more pills or blood pressure testing.

My friend explained that we each choose or decide everything either through our conscious or else our subconscious mind. Regardless where our thoughts arise, our subconscious will Intentionalize every aspect of how we manifest our body. She described how my mind was Intentionally creating what and how my body looked and felt.

"You have a choice!" she insisted.

She reminded me that I have dominion and control through my mind. This is a powerful Christian Science tenet which I readily grasped and could apply in the new awareness she was teaching me. Her confident understanding showed me that I could immediately make a change in how my body physically manifested. She emphasized that I was not getting all my symptoms from anything other than my self-imposed choice to believe that I'm just a frail body subject to ill health. She reminded me that I am not a frail body but an all-powerful mind and to take this knowledge and know it with Intentionality.

My friend explained to me the concept of ℒife Force that is used in *The Story of ℒife* book. How it flows through my body and mind full of healing energy, health, and wellness. She taught me to visualize it coming into my body, then flowing through it like a recycling fountain, flowing up and out to flow over my skin and then back into myself. Over and over, again and again. I pictured one of those beautiful water fountains in the park while I lay down or sat in a chair to bring it in and feel its energy. I learned to float in my ℒife Force consciously flowing through my body, relaxing and enjoying the confidence of my new understanding. In this way, I began to relax. To calm myself down when I was anxious, frightened, or uncomfortable, which very often I was. And my body followed my mind! My symptoms always lessened or went away.

Chris, the author of *The Story of ℒife*, included me in his healing group to heal my physical body even as Mina was healing my mind, what Chris' book calls the psyche, which includes much more than just my mere mind.

At last, I found myself walking a little farther each time. Freedom and fresh air! How glorious! I did have to be persistent with trusting Life [*Life capitalized is a Christian Science concept* —editor] and not let fears about heredity, aging, and so on creep into my thoughts. I found it easier to trust Life, to float in ℒife Force serene and calm . . . peaceful. Like floating on the water. Now I am able to walk mostly without my walking stick. Problems with digestion improved. My heart and breathing is making huge progress.

After about seven months I received a sum of money owed me by a relative, someone whom I thought had wronged me several years ago. I was able to contact this relative and forgive them, forget the past, and wish them well. I felt my resentment dissolve. This was a great burden lifted from my life. It's the healing that my friend talked about from *The Story of ℒife*.

In May, 2024 I was able to buy a used car in good condition for an affordable price. This was a real blessing since I had been without a car for so long. I'm now able to drive most of the time without any anxiety at all. I feel more calm, at ease, and relaxed and not so afraid and concerned about my health since I know that ℒife Force is flowing consciously through me and all around me, and is unstoppable.

I know there is no death of *me*, the person. It's impossible. My friend taught me how to talk with Mina through energy testing, which is discussed in the book, and I discovered not only him but also my deceased (spirit) family who are spending time with me to support my daily life. I can't express how incredibly healing that was for me to know!

Whenever I ever feel unwell or anxious, I ask Mina to heal me and protect me, and he always does. He helps me to let go of the fear of the unknown. *The Story of ℒife*, Chris, and my friend really made a difference for me. They helped me find much greater awareness of my own abilities using Intentionality to give me much better health. I am very grateful for the healing efforts of Chris and my friend in overcoming my fear and anxiety and how they were manifesting in my body. I give gratitude to Life and ℒife for all the blessings, healing, and spiritual progress in my life.

Scott

About 18 years ago I was diagnosed with an autoimmune disease called Myasthenia Gravis (MG). It is a disease where the muscles do not communicate correctly with the nerves, often attacking the face, eyes, or other parts of the body where there are sensitive muscles. At that time, my eyelids would not stay up by themselves. I experienced double vision as well as difficulty doing even simple things like swallowing. Driving was soon out of the question. MG is a relatively rare disease and I went to a whole host of doctors before finally receiving my diagnosis.

My doctor put me on steroids. I then graduated to some strong immune suppressants. One is Azathioprine, originally developed to prevent organ rejection after surgery. I have continued taking them for years to, at the very least, mitigate the worst of my symptoms. About two years ago, doctors asked me to consider a "breakthrough treatment" called Ultomiris, which they would administer through intravenous infusion about every eight weeks. After three or four treatments, their studies said that I could slowly eliminate my immune suppressant medications. Boy, were they wrong!

The symptoms came back fast after a few months worse than ever. My neurologist was genuinely sympathetic. All he could say was, "Yes, the treatment does not work for everyone."

"Thanks?"

In the meantime, I had lost more control of my arm and leg and stomach muscles. So much so that on one occasion I couldn't get out of the bathtub. Frequently, I couldn't take full breaths when lying down, or even roll over when I was sleeping in order to get a full breath. It was a very scary time for me every night. Absolutely terrifying! That fear is almost impossible to describe to anyone who hasn't experienced something like that—breath by breath by breath.

Anyway, I went back to taking the full dose of immune suppressants. Thankfully, many of the symptoms began to go away. But I still couldn't get back to zero point, the level I was at before that medical backslide. Then a new symptom appeared. I was now unable to move my jaw muscles with any force. I had a difficult time chewing and had to use my thumb to apply pressure whenever I would engage—or try to—my jaw muscles. Needless to say, I absolutely hated going out! I felt very, very self-conscious about this disability. I mostly only managed to eat soups and eggs. The one upside to all of this is that I lost a good amount of weight during this time simply through not eating.

Friends asked, "What's your secret?"

What could I say? I could only mouth, "Don't eat as much!" Yeah, not very inspiring.

Some visiting friends clued me in to Chris and his team. He was gracious enough to put me on his healing circle's list. I'm a very positive person . . . you have to be in my situation. I had to keep up my trust in new things howsoever they might come along into my life. Well, I am very grateful. He never asked me for anything in return. Slowly and surely my chewing problem began to diminish. Day after day I could feel a basic sense of happiness come back that I had been pushing down the last year. It makes me smile to think about being so happy about such a basic thing as chewing. Who knew?

And, it gets better. When I had recently gained about 60% of my chewing ability back, my friends gave me a message from Chris that I should expect to see a marked improvement in just the following three to four weeks. Guess what? I did! And right at the time which they told me he said it would happen. So much so that I'm now back to about 90% full chewing. Often I get through a whole meal now. Sometimes even including potato chips. Considering that just a year ago even cooked potatoes were off the table, it's wonderful to experience this now. What's more, it has led me to stop settling for bad health. I have noticed that I am pushing myself out of the house for longer walks every few days. I even put my step counter back on . . . and . . . all I can say is, "*We're back in business, folks!*" This is worth its weight in gold, believe me. I am deeply grateful to Chris' healing work.

Tony ✉

I'm 71 years old. Ever since I was 62 I have had problems with my prostate waking me up more and more at night for the bathroom. Finally, I was waking up every hour at night and quite often needed a bathroom even during the day. I read articles, watched YouTube videos, and researched the many ways that people promise to cure or, at the least, lessen it. My urologist diagnosed me with benign prostatic hyperplasia (BPH), which means an enlarged prostate. He wanted me to go the path of surgery but I couldn't resonate with that. I knew from my experiences talking to other men and family members that people who had surgery to remove or scrape their prostate usually didn't have good outcomes. After a lot of due diligence, I felt more comfortable with the naturopathic way as opposed to the allopathic way.

I watched many infomercials for prostate health that promised to cure me from waking up so often for the bathroom. Over the years, I tried at least a dozen of Amazon's miracle cures. The pills were expensive but didn't do much to alleviate the problem. This was so frustrating because they promised the world. But I was getting older and things only worsened. Naturally, I tried a wide variety of herbs, too. These included saw palmetto, stinging nettles, pygeum, and berries. They seemed to help a little but the problem didn't go away.

Finally, I came across *The Story of Life* and healing group. I asked if they could heal my prostate. The book's author, a spirit medium and Intentional healer, said it was caused by a spiritual attack as well as from my subconscious. He neutralized the cause and, very excitedly, I began my healing journey back toward health trusting in God it would work. It was a gradual process over several months. Little by little, I was waking up less and less. The period between waking up for the bathroom went from every single hour to two hours a night, then to three and four hours. After about three and a half months, I was waking up only once per night. Amazingly, some nights I didn't wake up at all!

I also learned that I need to remove my subconscious resistance to healing so that the condition would not return and my physical body would permanently heal. It was not easy to change my subconscious thinking since I wasn't even aware of it. I realized that I had buried, denied, or forgotten many traumas in my life from rejection, abandonment, failure, and a lack of love from my grandparents, parents, uncles, and aunts.

I had to ask Mina ('God') to help me let go of the low self-esteem, guilt, and feelings that I didn't deserve anything good. I thought I was supposed to suffer. Or at least sacrifice more to make all my problems less. It was a mind bending situation. I was caught between a rock and a hard place, as I was influenced by my religion and society to live according to their way of thinking, which turned out to be entirely not so beneficial let alone not useful. I didn't know what, much less how, to remove all the problematic thinking that was ingrained in my subconscious.

Well, I just started to work on myself, to accept what happened over the course of my life. I made a conscious choice to let go of the past memories causing me so much inner conflict that resulted in bad relationships, job losses, unresolved conflicts, and lack of confidence along with unwarranted fears and anxieties. It was like I had been sabotaging my own self. Or else something inside was holding me back from experiencing the good health and happiness I saw in Chris and others despite all the difficulties that had plagued their own lives over the years. But taking up *The Story of Life* and how it approached healing a person's body and mind was a big pill to swallow. In fact, I was not only afraid of what other people would think, but also what our judgmental Creator would think about it . . . and maybe judge me for.

I found out I couldn't let my pain and suffering go as easily as I'd imagined. I learned how to do the energy testing that Chris teaches in his book, which I'd practiced for years in a lesser form as 'muscle testing' for other reasons. Little by little, I felt my internal burden lighten up, even more so when I asked Mina through energy testing to help me understand what it was and to let it go. It felt like I'd won the lottery or found the combination that finally opened the right door.

All I can say is that it's miraculous. Mina just melted or removed the pain and it literally became just a memory and not a trigger or hot button that would set me off. I had no idea that our mind can not only hurt us but also heal us, or that so-called God (Mina) can help us heal if we only reach out and ask. There is a constant barrage of misinformation that we're supposed to get sick, disabled, or even die in a certain age range because of this or that situation. Even my hardened belief that my prostate was not working right simply because I was getting old was very strongly ingrained. I never realized that my mind was the remote cause of not only my mental and emotional problems but my actual physical problems, too. Through asking for healing and trying myself to let go of my inner conflicting issues, I am now on a better path to physical healing and spiritual awareness. Which is, needless to say, really important as you get older.

Harriet (P)

This testimony is long overdue because I have been running around with a heart full of gratitude for my physical activities including swimming, walking, gym classes, and yoga as well as pinochle and other card games, volunteer and other work as needed. All of this is normal for me, but had unexpectedly halted early in summer 2024 when I experienced an abnormal, slightly bloody discharge that didn't go away. Instead, it increased.

I applied my understanding of God and His creation as I have all my life as a Christian Scientist, having many physical healings over the years.

Although there wasn't much improvement at first, I wasn't concerned. I knew I didn't have to be impressed by physical symptoms. Just rely on the spiritual truth of God and His creation as I always have. I blocked all negative suggestions coming from my mind. However, the symptoms only strengthened. The "what ifs" started: what if it gets worse or doesn't stop? what if it's this or that? what if I don't get better? what caused it?

I continued using my Christian Science understanding of God and my identity as His child, but was not getting better. Then one morning I awoke with a stiff neck. I first thought I had slept in a wrong position but soon I saw it getting worse instead of better. I finally called my friend to help me pray to get on with a healing.

She had recently gained a new awareness in her lifelong understanding of creation and the universe through her reading *The Story of Life*. It gave her the needed perspective to more confidently help me. She suggested I join the healing group she was in with the author, which would give me the strong support I was desiring. Talking about her new awareness was so productive. An immediate, calm assurance poured forth like water flowing over the desert sand. I felt calmed in thought and the discharge lessened immediately. But the stiff neck got worse, and was quite painful.

The fear my family and I felt was difficult to overcome. I was drinking in every word she told me. She stressed that *Life* force was flowing through me like a recycling fountain that could not be interrupted. She gave me new ways to visualize this flowing river of *Life* force that never stops nor depletes. It is infinite, eternal, and is always healthy and complete. This really helped me obtain more confidence to change my thinking to lessen my fear. Her confidence that all healing happens because of awareness and that our own was growing every day gave me so much to rest on. I calmly knew that, no matter what physical appearances showed, I was healing mentally and it would manifest in my physical body.

The discharge lessened week by week but my neck turned into a very stiff and painful back. I was almost immobilized and needed help moving and getting out of bed. My fear kept me questioning my life as it worsened. It came to the point that, if I didn't get better soon, something would have to change. My family was more and more concerned and wanted me to see a doctor. They wanted to honor my faith in prayer for healing but were alarmed at my worsening condition. I agreed to check into a Christian Science nursing facility if I wasn't better soon. I prayed hard to do the right thing because I didn't want to further burden family. But I knew I would have a healing even though it seemed the opposite of my reality.

My friend reminded me that it was natural to feel *Life* force constantly flowing through and around me. She said I can feel it and know it with confidence. My health, happiness, freedom, joy, harmony, living, moving—all are eternal and strong since they exist in my *Life* force flowing constantly and consistently. It never stops nor is impeded. Nothing can disrupt it. I knew it but had trouble confidently feeling it despite reminding myself hourly and daily suffering in bed.

I didn't want to leave my home, and it didn't seem to me that I should have to change my physical location to experience healing. My friend calmly, yet strongly reassured me that I couldn't make a wrong decision. That if I needed to go someplace for physical care, I could do so without feeling bad about my decision or upsetting the healing process.

I called a local nursing facility. They very soothingly assured me that a room was available if I needed care. While I prayed, they comforted my granddaughter that I'd have proper care. My granddaughter felt greatly relieved that they wouldn't leave a patient to waste away in bed all the time. My family's concerns were lovingly, completely answered. It alleviated their fears.

My friend's loving, steadfast support with the author's healing group, and her awareness of *Life* force from *The Story of Life* and its constant flowing and infinitude, helped me let go of my fear and to leave it all to *Life* force to sustain my physical body as well as to mentally stop resisting the healing that was happening in my body. Within the next couple of days, I felt great physical and mental improvement. I had let go of the physical body problems as a part of my being and completely let *Life* force flow without interference from my thinking. My friend and her healing group made a big difference in this healing that I had. I understand my *Life* force more completely and have more confidence in it for my own health and well being.

Gratitude, gratitude, gratitude. So very grateful for the absolute steadfastness, dedication and constant availability and immediate comfort and encouragement. It all seems like a bad dream now.

I didn't realize until after the healing how subtle human fear can be as it raised up names of fearful diseases. How some symptoms suggest ideas of age making me more vulnerable, that we are naturally having more physical problems that we can't overcome. Or suggesting that Intentional thinking about *Life* force doesn't always heal everything. Or that maybe my work here is done and no one lives forever. That maybe I should be willing to accept what might come . . . *yada, yada, yada.* ALL LIES!

I returned to all my activities in about a month after joining the healing group. I feel ℒife force flowing through me all the time. It doesn't stop and neither do I! I am joyfully accepting ℒife lovingly flowing over me.

Amelia (P)

Growing up—and until I noticed bald patches in September or October 2020—I had long, thick, lustrous hair. It was my pride and joy. I never imagined my hair could or would fall out of my head. It was a heart wrenching shock! I think my father's death in July of 2020 triggered it. Losing him left me completely heartbroken, just devastated.

I went to my primary doctor. She diagnosed me with alopecia and referred me to a dermatologist. They gave me steroid shots in my scalp to stimulate hair growth. But when I left the office that day, I was extremely sick with a headache and wanted to vomit. I had to lay down the remainder of the day. I couldn't even take care of my four boys who were ages 2, 4, 6, and 7 years old.

The steroids didn't work and I didn't continue the treatment, partly because it made me so sick. I tried topical treatments. I qualified for clinical trials for hair growth oral medication and had a little hair growth, but they stopped it because my hair recovery wasn't good enough. I felt defeated and gave up hope of ever having hair again . . . of being a bald woman the rest of my life.

Then through a friend, the author of *The Story of ℒife* book, Chris, added me to his healing group in July 2023. He started working on my hair and immediately it started to grow! It was growing back fast and furious and was very strong and stable when I tugged on it. I had nearly a full head of hair maybe three inches long by March of 2024.

Unfortunately, I noticed in April that I was getting bad psoriasis. It was causing me to pick at my scalp and pull out my hair. By mid April, I got word of two very difficult life events that put me into a severe depression. My hair started falling out again. I ended up with a completely bald head for the entirety of the summer. As I successfully coped with my new depression, I once again saw hair growth in August 2024, though this time it's been fragile and thin.

Through *The Story of ℒife* and talking with its author, Chris, I've been learning to cope with depression and life's travails without letting my emotional state manifest poor health such as my hair loss. He has taught me how to control and understand my empath experiences that I have had for my whole life without ever understanding it. *The Story of ℒife* explains what happens when an empath experiences others' emotions and what we can do to relieve ourselves of these strong emotions that overwhelm us. He taught me about neutralizing the energy around me and my family that makes us sick or puts us in turmoil.

Psyche Healing

I learned about the energy that influences us when Chris made me aware of the energy of an individual who was very angry at our family for the past two-plus years with no apology in sight. That anger, as negative emotive ℒife force, was making our family physically sick and causing my children and me to experience many harmful events. Chris included this person in his psyche healing group with their spirit self's permission. Within 10 months of this inclusion, this person openly apologized to our family literally out of the blue for their actions and attitude. It was a remarkable turn of events for this person and us. We all continue to heal from the long-term effects of that negative EMℒF as well as the negative Intentionality that directly harmed us. I am more than grateful for this huge healing for our family!

Matoka

In January, 2024 our dog, Matoka, was limping and protectively barking very aggressively at people who came to visit. Her limping was from knee injuries arising in her first three years of life before coming to us. We believe she was used for dog fighting but aren't sure; she has definite scars from fighting other dogs. Chris added her to his healing group and within a few weeks she'd stopped limping and was becoming so much calmer and much less agitated. She is a new dog.

I am learning how to recognize the energy that effects us. Through Chris' mentoring, I am able to understand better how to help my family and the healing process in both my psyche and physical body. With my hair regrowth and experience healing my emotions so far, I'm confident not only my family but this other person and my hair, too, will make a complete recovery as we all continue healing inside.

Join our free healing group at chrismckeon.com/healing-group.

Thank you for reading my story! Would you leave a review for others who might benefit? It means a lot to me. Your support makes a difference; I read all reviews for feedback to make my books even better. Just follow the link (https://books2read.com/yourbodybook).

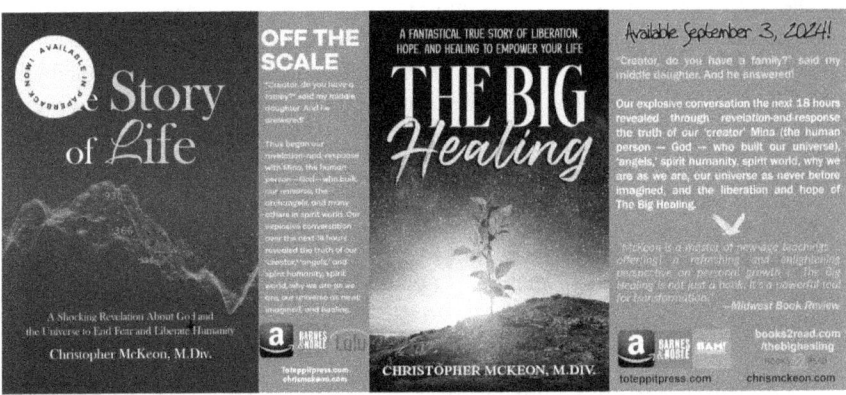

The Big Healing is the exciting first 10 chapters of *The Story of Life*'s total 42 chapters.

 SoL Hardcover ☞ Paperback ☞ FREE Kindle

 TBH Hardcover ☞ Paperback ☞ Kindle/ePub

Turn the page to read a sample from Chapter 1: "All Shook Up"

Thursday October 12, 2017 ca. 5 PM

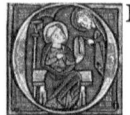**F ALL THE** days in all the months in all the year, Friday the 13th just had to be the day the world as it was all sort of just blew up in our face. My two daughters and I . . . well, we quite lit the fuse when, about sixteen hours before that cool October morning, we'd tramped through the garage door of our woodsy rural log cabin home following an afternoon of errands and posed a simple question. Atop a wild, spiritually hectic week culminating in our long afternoon in the car talking over God, ancestry, life, and surprises from dear dead friends, my two-days-eighteen daughter El froze mid-step in our living room and blurted, "Creator, do you have a family?"

And he answered.

We all three traded surprised eyes at the *yes* response, but she was on a roll.

"Do you have a wife?"

Yes.

"Do you have children, not just us?"

Yes.

She paused a few seconds, thinking through the logic. "Do you have a *mother?*"

Yes!

While I jacked my jaw up off the floor, she looked at me. "Dad, I can literally *feel* his joy that we've just discovered this! He's really happy! Can we meet her?" she added, not to me. "Can we talk to her?"

At which point El swiveled to her right, face and eyes cranking upward as though at a much taller person. Her expression transformed, aglow with delight and excitement. A smile burst across her cheeks as her hands flew to her heart. She sucked her breath.

"*Hi*, Mother!"

Yeah. I gawped, too.

Even a wizened skeptic like me could tell my younger daughter was having a moment, an experience, a—well, a revelation. Chills, tingles, and heat shivered me timbers stem to stern. Energy and pleasure radiated from El. I could see her gleam. There was no mistaking her profound joy and rapture. We, too, felt the presence of 'Mother' fiercely blazing with happy excitement. Communicating. In our *home*. To *us*. Who were *aware* of her. My older daughter and resident spiritualist Ayako, now two days from her twenty-first year, twisted round a blue-upholstered, high-backed dining chair and plopped into it facing El with a knowing curiosity, feeling all the energy we were experiencing and more. We incessantly questioned Mother and Mina—God—into the night, all of which you'll encounter throughout this book.

That wasn't even the really exciting part. But before we got to that, our curiosity slanted us through some scary hours later in the night that left my exuberant daughters tearful and terrified, and me wondering just what can of worms we'd pulled the pop-top on. For now, though, we enthusiastically pushed our envelope of reality and the eye-popping responses snowballed. A lifelong Irish Roman Catholic, Protestant Christian, Unificationist, and now post-Unificationist, it soon registered that my worldview, my *lifeview*, was in some real distress here. Stuff needed clarifying if not a little unmitigated arguing. Yet for all that, Mina's answers were coherent, consistent, and sensible. Only good, loving, calm but excited energy bathed the room. With that, it seemed as wise a time as any to get down to the suddenly apropos nitty-gritty.

I said, "Creator, is the Bible true?"

No.

I pulled a hard breath, astonished, though as a graduate of divinity school maybe not all that surprised. Even so, a linchpin of my lifeview clattered to the wide-planked floor.

"What about the New Testament? Is Jesus' teaching in that true?"

"Dad, he said—"

No.

"*All* of it?" I gave my girls each a once over, but if you could wear a body shrug like a pantsuit, they were. *Kids*, I thought. Always jaunty at the start of a march across somebody else's Bataan.

No.

"So, some of it, then, is true."

Yes.

"How 'bout Jesus," El said, "is he a real person?"

Yes.

Well, that was a relief. I think. Anyhow, the girls looked copacetic. We quizzed Mina on this topic awhile until, inevitably, it led to the issue most pressing me.

"Is Rev. Moon's teaching in *Divine Principle* true?" I mean, I'd largely bet the farm on it in 1981.

No.

My ribs fell in. There went another linchpin. I let out a wheeze like I'd just downed a shot of two-hundred proof. Bleary eyes landed on each daughter, but saw in them none of my own jolt.

"Jeez, girls," I yawped. "That's been my lifeview purt' near forty years!"

Ever sassy, Ayako said, "Welcome to the next wave, Dad."

Unlike Jesus, I *knew* Sun-myung (he eschews titles, now). His theologically ultra-modern Divine Principle was more real to me than worn out, foggy old Christianity, its grand morsels of wisdom and Jesus notwithstanding. Sure, Divine Principle reposed upon the biblical witness, but to me it more sensibly elucidated its core truths. It underwrote the full scale of my adult life. I might be perennially at war with Sun-myung's pigheaded church institution but not his Divine Principle, not by any stretch.

I said, "*All* of it?"

I had to ask because, like everyone in spirit world communicating with a non-conversational medium in the physical world, Mina must needs be literal in our mode of communication. He has to be, really. Absent face-to-face or even just voice-to-voice conversation, it's nigh impossible to gauge what a person actually means by words alone. Consider how the misunderstanding curve rises proportionally to one's metaphorical distance from the speaker. One's words themselves—rooting in shared definitions—need convey precisely what's meant. That's a tough row to hoe for humans, wedded the way we are to contextual word play. You might think Mina could simply know our thoughts, but that creates complications of its own we discuss later. What it boils down to, Ayako pointed out, is that we had to formulate our questions thoughtfully into unambiguous inquiries and confirmations that backed up our responses.

No, Mina answered me through El.

Huh. So again, only some of my lifeview was true. Was that good? I didn't know. As with the Bible, I could only wonder, *which freaking part? Divine Principle* is a weighty *vade mecum* in its own right.

Being young, unformed, and like many in their generation rejecting religion generally though not God specifically, my daughters *looked* okay—my eldest like an old soul hearing something she'd long suspected and her kid sister charmed in high cotton—but *my* cosmology was melting apart like Icarus' wishful wax job. This conversation was sweeping away a lifetime of hard-won truths, from the nature of the universe and God to Jesus and Sun-myung's messianism and the spiritual verity and providential histories that went with them (likewise with all religions), not to mention what I'd sacrificed—wasted?—for it all. My head was spinning. I was anything *but* okay. But dammitall if that would throttle my interest; perish the thought. Come hell or high water, I'm nothing if not the cat tempting curiosity.

By and by, we worked our way to the crux of the Abrahamic religions: the Fall of Man. Original sin territory and their *raison d'être*. After some unexpected and perplexing responses from Mina, we needed to get a few things straight.

I said, "Are you saying the Fall never happened?"

Yes.

"So . . ." dittoed El, finally sounding a tad betrayed, "there *was* no Fall of Man?"

No.

"Satan never persuaded Eve to eat the 'fruit'?" she continued. "Lucifer never fell—never had a wrong sexual relationship with Eve like Rev. Moon said? People never tried to be God and 'fell' from grace or perfection, or whatever?"

No, no, no.

"Well," said I, "fuuu—!"

No.

Ayako shifted round to me with disapprobation. "That 'no' means negative energy resonates, Dad."

Great.

After more give-and-take—during which Mina recast 'the Fall' as *The Corruption* in which humans self-manifested our selfish, harmful world and self-alienated ourselves from God (I mean, Mina) without any help from anybody, including our evolutionarily left-over, full-blown-batty reptile brain—El perceptively said, "Wait. Are Adam and Eve even real people who actually lived?"

No.

Ayako and El traded stares. It seemed their own lifeviews were at last meeting some unexpected renovation. About time.

I choked. "Um, they don't exist?"

No. They don't exist.

"Then, is Satan a real being, a fallen angel, or . . . whatever?"

No. No . . . no.

"Wait, wait." Just. *Wait*. I needed a minute to *think*.

El didn't. "You mean Satan doesn't even *exist*? There's no devil, no evil force or being that—"

No, no.

"So, no war in heaven, no angel rebellion, no beings cast down to earth," she went on with obvious offense, practically ticking through Revelations (12:7–9) on her fingers and giving me, her ministerial, semi-Bible-thumping father a flinty eye, "no ancient good versus . . . *none* of these stories religion taught us are true?"

No. Sorry.

El blew off a heavy breath, threw up her hands, and tromped in a circle. Oaths welled up in my brain so fast they had to take a number.

A little hostile, I said, "What about Darwin, then?"

"Not Darwin, Dad," said Ayako, ever the schoolteacher, "Darwin*ism*. Unless you mean the guy, you're talking about natural selection."

"Uh, sure . . . but is he—it—true?"

No.

"What? But then—?"

"So, evolution is *wrong*?" said El.

Yes.

"All of it?" I added, pretty much expecting the obvious.

No.

Yep. Here we go again. "So, basically, *everybody's* explanation for humanity's existence and miserable condition is total bullshit?"

"Dad . . ."

"False?"

Maybe . . . yes.

Ayako said, "Remember, Dad, he said not *every* single thing."

"Yeah, but everybody's?"

"Like, all religions and philosophies?" El said plainly.

Yes.

She let out a low, gruff whistle. "*Waaah*—when your whole existence is just a fat lie."

"So, Islam, too?" I said. "And Buddhism, Confucianism, Hinduism, Animism—"

Yes, yes, ye—

Ayako gave me an eye. "He said all religions, Dad. Come on."

Yes.

"I'm just being thorough." And not taking sides, I didn't say.

No.

"I'm not? But I . . . wait," I said toward El, who was doing our energy testing. "Are you pulling my leg?"

Yes.

"Well. Isn't he just a barrel of monkeys. Never took God for a joker," I said to Ayako, though I'd heard a medium once make the claim.

"Lots of things you never thought of, Dad," she chirped, queen of the snappy comeback and earning my tight-lipped stare-down. My mood was a little nettled, frankly.

A flurry of questions and statements followed as we plunged ever deeper down our rabbit hole. I put evolution aside for now. It only dealt with our bodies anyhow. We had *cosmic* issues on the table. But now, a few other things in my head about the human 'fall from grace' were rising to the fore and clashing with Mina's assertions. It occurred to me we'd need to pull in somebody else, the very somebody who off and on since late summer had purveyed through a local medium a seemingly clear, unambiguous spiritual reality that included a very real Adam and Eve. Archangel Michael.

Read the rest of

The Big Event in . . .

The Big Healing

wherever books are sold;

or get the full monty including ALL EXISTENCE, ALL THAT'S IN IT, AND US, and ENERGY TESTING plus ten spirit world testimonies from historical figures including Jesus, Sun-myung Moon, Mohammad, Buddha, and Hitler in

The Story of Life

Hardcover, paperback, and *free* eBook (at select locations) wherever books are sold.

Use your smartphone camera to follow the QR codes below to (L–R) visit the author at chrismckeon.com, visit toteppitpress.com for a *free* PDF with clickable cross-reference links, purchase *The Story of Life* (or download *free* Kindle), or purchase *The Big Healing*. Thank you!

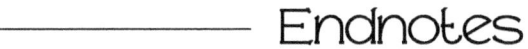

Endnotes

1. (page 51)   Source: *left* [modified to inverted b/w] https://www.shutterstock.com/video/clip-710974-multicolored-balls-floating-inflatable-water-pool; *right* [modified to b/w] https://aeo1.alicdn.com/kf/HTB14PRVd25TBuNjSspmq6yDRVXa7/New-Toy-2018-Human-Bubble-Ball-Inflatable-Walk-On-Water-Ball-For-Swimming-Pool-Floating-Walking.jpg (accessed: 2024-11-22).
2. (page 74)   Sofie Jackson "Humans do have a SIXTH SENSE: Scientists in bombshell brainwaves claim," from https://www.dailystar.co.uk/news/latest-news/magnetic-field-humans-magnetoreception-sixth-17131664 (accessed 2024-11-25).

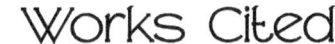
Works Cited

Explanatory Note: Works cited form no part (though some coincidentally agree in part with the text) of this book beyond short quotes or as a reference. They represent background material that informed and guided our ET inquiries in areas where our awareness was deficient.

American Heritage Dictionary of the English Language. 2020. 5th ed. Boston: Houghton Mifflin Harcourt Publishing Company. [cit. 99].

Bandura, Albert. 1963. *Social Learning and Personality Development.* NY: Holt, Rinehart, and Winston. [cit. 88].

Bandura, Albert. 1986. *Social Foundations of Thought and Action: A Social Cognitive Theory.* NY: Prentice-Hall. [cit. 88].

Bandura, Albert. 1995. *Self-efficacy in changing societies.* NY: Cambridge Univ. Press. [cit. 88].

Bandura, Albert. 1997. *Self-efficacy: The exercise of control.* NY: W.H. Freeman. [cit. 88].

Cambridge English Dictionary. 2022. Cambridge, UK: Cambridge Univ. Press. [cit. 29–30].

Chalmers, David J. 2006. "Strong and Weak Emergence." In *The Re-Emergence of Emergence: The Emergentist Hypothesis from Science to Religion,* 244–56. Oxford Univ. Press. [cit. 27].

Cianciolo, Anna T., and Robert J. Sternberg. 2004. *Intelligence: A Brief History.* Malden, MA: Blackwell Publishing. [cit. 30].

Clayton, Philip. 2006. "Conceptual Foundations of Emergence Theory." In *The Re-Emergence of Emergence: The Emergentist Hypothesis from Science to Religion,* edited by Paul Davies and Philip Clayton, 1–34. Oxford University Press. [cit. 27].

Davies, Paul. 2007. *Cosmic Jackpot: Why Our Universe is Just Right for Life.* NY: Houghton Mifflin. [cit. 29].

De Wolf, Tom, and Tom Holvoet. 2005. "Emergence Versus Self-Organisation: Different Concepts but Promising When Combined," edited by Sven A. Brueckner, Giovanna Di Marzo Serugendo, Anthony Karageorgos, and Radhika Nagpal, 3464:1–15, July 25, 2004. Utrecht, The Netherlands: Springer. https://doi.org/10.1007/b136984. [cit. 27].

Dumper, Kathryn, William Jenkins, Arlene Lacombe, Marilyn Lovett, and Marion Perimutter. 2019. *Introductory Psychology: What is Cognition?* Edited by Samantha Swindell. Open Text Washington State University. Accessed March 30, 2020. https://opentext.wsu.edu/psych105/chapter/7-2-what-is-cognition/. [cit. 30].

Eddy, Mary Baker. 1896. *Miscellaneous Writings: 1883–1896.* Boston, MA: The Trustees under the Will of Mary Baker G. Eddy. [cit. 186].

Gottfredson, Linda S. 1997. "Mainstream science on intelligence: An editorial with 52 signatories, history, and bibliography." Originally published in *The Wall Street Journal* December 13, 1994. *Intelligence* 24, no. 1 (January–February): 13–23. Accessed February 14, 2019. https://doi.org/10.1016/S0160-2896(97)90011-8. [cit. 30].

Green, Douglas R., Lorenzo Galluzzi, and Guido Kroemer. 2014. "Metabolic control of cell death." *Science* 345, no. 6203 (September 19, 2014): 1466. [cit. 54–55].

Hartwell, Leland H., and Ted A. Weinert. 1989. "Checkpoints: Controls that Ensure the Order of Cell Cycle Events." *Science* 246, no. 4930 (November 3, 1989): 629–634. [cit. 53–55].

Henriques, Gregg. 2011. "What is the Mind? Understanding mind and consciousness via the unified theory." In *Psychology Today.* December 22, 2011. Accessed April 29, 2020. https://www.psychologytoday.com/us/blog/theory-knowledge/201112/what-is-the-mind. [cit. 70].

Holman, Peggy. 2010. *Engaging Emergence: Turning Upheaval Into Opportunity.* San Francisco: Berrett-Koehler. [cit. 26–27].

Hunt, Tim, Kim Nasmyth, and Béla Novák. 2011. "The cell cycle." *Philosophical Transactions: Biological Sciences* 366, no. 1584 (December 27, 2011): 3494–3497. [cit. 53].

Works Cited

Huxley, Julian. 1942. *Evolution: The Modern Synthesis*. NY: Harper & Brothers. [cit. 43].

Johnson, Steven. 2001. *Emergence: The Connected Lives of Ants, Brains, Cities, and Software*. NY: Scribner. [cit. 27].

Lewis, Ralph M.D. 2023. "How Could Mind Emerge From Mindless Matter." Adapted from *Finding Purpose in a Godless World: Why We Care Even If The Universe Doesn't* (Amherst, NY: Prometheus Books, 2018), *Psychology Today* (October 7, 2023). Accessed December 1, 2024. https://www.psychologytoday.com/us/blog/finding-purpose/201901/how-could-mind-emerge-from-mindless-matter. [cit. 2].

Lovelock, John. 1979. *Gaia: A New Look at Life on Earth*. Oxford University Press. [cit. 28].

Mancuso, Stefano, and Alessandra Viola. 2015. *Brilliant Green: The Surprising History and Science of Plant Intelligence*. Wash. DC: Island Press. [cit. 30].

McKeon, Christopher. 2022. *The Story of Life: A Shocking Revelation About God and the Universe to End Fear and Liberate Humanity*. Rico, CO: Tōteppit Press. [cit. i, 1].

McKeon, Christopher. 2024. *The Big Healing: A Fantastical True Story of Liberation, Hope, and Healing to Empower Your Life*. Rico, CO: Tōteppit Press. [cit. i, 7].

Merriam-Webster Dictionary. 2022. Springfield, MA: Encyclopædia Britannica. [cit. 10, 140].

O'Connor, Timothy. 1994. "Emergent Properties." *Amer Phil Qtrly* 31, no. 2 (April): 91–104. Accessed February 5, 2019. https://www.jstor.org/stable/20014490. [cit. 27].

O'Connor, Timothy, and Hong Yu Wong. 2015. "Emergent Properties." In *The Stanford Encyclopedia of Philosophy*, Summer, edited by Edward N. Zalta. Metaphysics Research Lab, Stanford University. https://plato.stanford.edu/entries/properties-emergent/. [cit. 27].

Parise, André Geremia, Monica Gagliano, and Gustavo Maia Souza. 2020. "Extended cognition in plants: is it possible?" *Plant Signaling & Behavior* 15 (2): 1710661. https://doi.org/10.1080/15592324.2019.1710661. [cit. 30].

Piiroinen, Tero. 2014. "Three Senses of 'Emergence': On the Term's History, Functions, and Usefulness in Social Theory." *Prolegomena* (Zagreb) 13 (1): 141–61. [cit. 26].

Rackham, Harris, trans. (c. 353–322 BC) 1956. *The Nicomachean Ethics*. By Aristotle. Edited by T.E. Page, E. Capps, W.H.D. Rouse, L.A. Post, and E.H. Warmington. Cambridge: Harvard University Press (Loeb Library Edition). [cit. 68].

Rosenbaum, Ernest H. MD, and Isadora R. Rosenbaum MA. 2024. "The Will to Live." Originally published in *Coping with Cancer*, March/April 1999, *Stanford Medicine Surviving Cancer*, accessed December 10, 2024. https://med.stanford.edu/survivingcancer/cancers-existential-questions/cancer-will-to-live.html. [cit. 126].

Rousseau, Jean-Jacques. 1761. *Discourse Upon the Origin and Foundation of the Inequality among Mankind*. London: R. & J. Dodsley, Pallmall. [cit. 6].

Sahni, Varun. 2002. "The cosmological constant problem and Quintessence." *Classical and Quantum Gravity* 19, no. 13 (June 12, 2002): 3435–48. https://doi.org/10.1088/0264-9381/19/13/304. [cit. 29].

Siegel, Daniel J. 2016. *Mind: A Journey to the Heart of Being Human*. NY: W.W. Norton. [cit. 70].

Tompkins, Peter, and Christopher Bird. 1973. *The Secret Life of Plants*. NY: Harper & Row. [cit. 30, 120].

Yildiz, A. 2024. "Mechanism and Regulation of Kinesin Motors." *Nat Rev Mol Cell Biol* (October 11, 2024). Accessed December 6, 2024. https://doi.org/10.1038/s41580-024-00780-6. [cit. 75].

Zlatev, Ivaylo, Limin Wang, and Paul J. Steinhardt. 1999. "Quintessence, Cosmic Coincidence, and the Cosmological Constant." *Physical Review Letters* 82:896–99. [cit. 29].

Index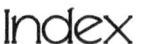

Bold page numbers indicate an entry's definitive reference(s) or is otherwise important. Some entries represent a range (e.g., biology [biological]; emergent [emergence]), others do double duty (e.g., biology for chemistry, biochemistry, etc.).

──────────────── ⊷୧❦୨⊶ ────────────────

Accountableism, 12, 15, **88–89**, 104, 106, 135, 164, 171, *see also* Corruption, The
   addiction to, 12, 164, 170, 174, 177, 181, 182
   altruism, **13**, 104, 182
addiction, *see* Accountableism; mindset
aging, 3, 9, 69, 88, 105, 112, 114, 117, 122, **123**, **125–126**, 132, 147, 159, 163, **167**, 174, 175, 187
'All there infinitely is', *see* All Existence
All Existence, 2, 4, 6, 11–13, 19, 20, **25–26**, 27–32, **33**, 35, **45**, 48, 50, 57, 59, 62, 81, 83–86, 90, 97, 98, 104, 113, 131, 135, 144, 145, 182
   analogy as primitive sea, **50–51**
   principal aspects, 11, **31**, 32–34
   self-aware, 3, **64**, 80
   'subconscious', 29
amalgamation, *see* mind ⌊subconscious
animal, 5, 7, 9, 18, 32, 70, 71, 73, 78, 89, 96, 103, 106, **119**, 120–123, 127, 132, 144, 147, 160, 161, 164, 168, *see also* nonhuman
   brain, 73, 109, 155, 156
   lifespans, 125
archí, 16–18, 20, 39, 50, 51, 58, 63, **66–67**, 81, 101, 111, 142, 162, 166
   analogy as air bubbles, 67
   analogy to ℒife, **36**
   force, 61, 141, 178
   pairwise, 20
astral projection, 7, 11, 17
attack, *see* spirit attack
autonomy, 4, 6, 29, 76, 135, 141, 186
   absolute, 3, 5, 7, **8**, 10, 12, 13, 18, 39, 45, 52, 107, 117, 134, **170**, **181**, 182
   non-, 12, 13, 89, 164, 181
aware
   self, 11, 98, 141
   un-, 12, **30**, 46, 64, 80, 97, 122, **125**, 139–141, 152, 158, 176, 178, 190
awareness, 5, 10, **18**, 24, **32**, 33, **41**, 47, **51**, **80**, **82**, **85**, **98**, **102**, **105**, 106, 107, 115, **118**, 120, 137, 138, **139–140**, 146, 147, 153, 158, 168, **173**, **176**, 177, 179, 182, 187, 194, *see also* self-awareness
   brain, 76, 109
   co-, twixt EPL & biology, 54, 56
   conscious, 10–12, 24, 109, 140, 158, 170

   % of wholistic mind, 136
   –experience, 6, 7, 9, 112, 144, 146, 147, 150, 152, 153, 156, 193, 194
   focal, 99, 154, 156, 194
   full, 14, **109**, 110, 120, 121, 147, 171, **182**
   mind, generally, 11, 30, 84, 85, 96, 109, 111, 121
   mode of, 77, 98, 121
   physicospirit, 79, 164
   spirit-aware, 18, 78
   state(s) of, **71**, 73, 74, 77, 98–100, 109–111, **120**, 121, 150, 155, 177, 179, 193, 194
   macro-, 73, 75
   micro-, 71, 73, 75, 76
   subconscious, 12, 77, 98–100, 102–104, 110, 112, 121, 155
   un, 141
   un-, 13, 30, 64, 71, 78–80, 82, 85, 106, 144, 148, 175, 177, 182, 190
   nonconscious intelligence, 27–29
   unlocks power of mind, 83
awareness–experiential, *see also* thinking–feeling; Thought

being, 29, 80, *see* self-aware proto-energy
   -ness, 32, 111, 113, 145, **152**, 164
   self-aware-, **97**, 99
   mode of, **28**, 51
   of mind, 72, 78
   state(s) of, **71**, 73–75, 77, 97–100, 103, 109–111, **120**, 121, 122, **124**, 135, 150, 165, 177, 179, 193, 194
   micro-, 73
belief, *vii*, 12, 13, 103, 114, 122, **162**, 167, 171, 173
   conscioius, 132
   conscious, 9
'belief', *see* mind ⌊subconsious
'belief', 122
Big Bang, *see* universe
Big Healing, 96, 101, 125, 135, **142**, 170, 175, 178, 182
biology, 5, 8, 9, 30, 38, 43, 47–50, 53–55, 80, 82, 83, 90, 91, 98, 101, 105, 114, 117, 121, 122, 124, 129–132, 135, 147, 148, 150, 162, 164, 166, 167, 171, 174, 175, 192, *see also* energy
   example: plant a flower, 65
biology, biological, 1

birth, 171, *see* emergence
    emergent, *see also* emergence
body, *see* embodiment
brain, 5, 8, 30, 49, 70–79, 89, 98, 99, 101, 109, 110, 121, 127, 130, 133, 138, 141, 142, **153**, 154–158, 161, 174, 191
    –body, 18, 70, 71, 77, 110
    –mind, 70
    -state, 77, 135, 155
    an electrochemical processor, 75
    animal, 73, 109, 155, 156
    body, 70
    human, 7, 9, 18, 57, 70, **72–79**
        an electrochemical processor, 72
    transliteration, **75**, 76, 77

chakras, 18, 124, **156**, **192–194**
    'energy', **193**
    aura, 193, 194
    closed, **193**
    energy, **192–194**
    'frequency'-resonance, 194
    open, **194**
coax, *see* Intentionality
conception, 1, 6, 7, 9, 10, 12, 24, 32, 52–54, 86, 113, 118, 131, 152, 162, 164, 173
conscious, 28, 29, 50, 53, **64**, 103, 109, *see also* mind ⌊conscious
    -ness, 24, 27, 29–32, **33**, 41, **42**, 51, **52**, 59, 71, **79–81**, 82, 83, 85, 90, 96–98, **117**, 120, 155
    non-, 29, 31, 50, 52, 90, 136, 154, 156, 159
consciousness, *see* psyche
Corruption, The, 10, **12–13**, 15, 38, 78, 89, **104–107**, 132, 135, 148, 170, 171, 178
    'energy' of, **107–109**
    interference of, 12, **13**, 76, **77**, 80, 88, **101**, 104–106, 121, 144, 153, 155, 159, 164, 175, 179, 181
culture, 38, 88, 89, 116, 122, **135**
    Ultimaculture, 135
    Ultraculture, 14, 89, 116, 122, **131**, 132, **134–136**, 166, 183

damage, 5, 72, 78, 81, 102, 103, 106, 108, 114, **118**, 120, **121**, 122, 126, 127, 130, 159, 163, 164, 167, 168, **169**, 170, 172–174, 176–180, 182, 185, 186, 190, *see also* 'energy'
    chronic, *v*, 123, 161, **168**, 169, 186, 188
    'energy' of, 120, 122, 134, 186, 188, 189
death, *v*, 1, 5, 10, 13, 56, 71, 88, 91, 103, 105–107, **126–127**, 132, 144, 147, 159, 165

embodied, *see* embodiment

embodiment, 11, 15, 32, 44, 79, 84, 85, **96**, 103, 135, 160, 189
    physical, 1–5, 7, 9–12, **14**, 15, 18, 24, 32, 37–39, 45, **46–47**, 57, 66, 69, 73, 74, 76, 80, 82, 83, 85, 86, 89–91, 96, 105, 113, 114, 119, 130, 131, 144, **152**, **163**, 164, 165, **170**, **171**, 178, 193
    archetype, 38, 47
physicospirit, 12, 78, 82, 130, 133
'reflective', 19, 186, 187, 193
    -self, 18
spirit, 3, 7–10, 12, 17–20, 33, 38, **45**, 48, 49, 76, 83–85, 91, 96, 106, 120, 129, 133, 149, **152**
spirit-born, 7
    un-, 38, 47, 48, 84, 85, 91, 135, 137
    analogy to sensory deprivation tank, 48
embryo, 54–56, 101
emergence
    weak, 73
emergent, **2**, 11, 20, **26–27**, 29, 32, **35**, **49**, 90, **113**, 141, 183, *see also* Way of Being
    birth, 1, 4, 7, 9, 10, 12, 24, 27, 31, 32, 37, 38, 45, **48**, 49, 52, 80–82, 86, 90, 97, 104, 111, 113, 114, 122, 129, 131, 143, 152, 164, 167, 173, 178, 181
    Intentionally triggered, 1, **2**, **47**, 48, 49, 52, 143
    Phase 1, 54
    Phase 2, **54–55**
    Phase 3, 53, **55**
    physical context, **53–56**
coalesce, 2, **36**, 50, 53, 113
differentiate, 2, **36**, 50, 53, 113
person, *see* person
property, 2, 3, 5, 31, 32, 71, 73, 81, 90
    examples, 73
proto-energy, **3**, 4, 5, 29, 108, 120, 126, **171**
proto-life, 7
self, 97, 101, **102**, 108, 111, 112, 117–120, 123, 126, 127, 129, **130**, 131–135, 140, 141, **152**, 154–159, 162, 165–169, 172, 173, 176, 180, 183, 186–188
    'energy of', 101–103, 130, **131**, 167
self-aware All Existence, 3
self-aware proto-energy, *see* self-aware proto-energy
self-organize, 2, 27, 29, **36**, 40, 52–54, 70, 88, 90, 113
strong, **27**, 73
Way of Being, *see* Way of Being
weak, **27**, 36, 60, 67, 71
Em⌊F, *see* emotive ⌊ife force
emotive ⌊ife force, 40, 110, 113, **123–125**, 135
    negative, 13, 14, **124–125**, 138, 151, **174**,

Index

175–178, **179**, 180–182
emotive energy, *see* emotive ℒife force
empath, 14, 123, **125**
encounter, 74, 76, 90, **96**, 100, 102, 115, **174**, 177, 188, 190
enérgeia, 66, *see* 'energy'
Energent, 2, 8, 9, 15, 16, 18, 19, 32, 45, **59–62, 66, 68**, 71, 81
 –prime, 2, 9–11, 19, 20, 31, 32, **33**, 35, 45, 50, 52, 54, **59–60, 65, 67**, 80–82, 131, 137, **138**, 141
 intelligence, **27–30**
 analogy as ocean energies, 60
 natural, 16–20, 52, 61, 62, 141, 148, 178, 186
 –prime, 178
 proto-energy, 2, 3, 7–9, **10**, 14–17, **19**, 32, 35, 52, **65, 66**, 71, 73, 75, 76, 80, **84**, 103, 104, **106**, 111, 113, 115, 123, 124, 131, 133, 135, 137, 141, 142, **145**, 149, 154, 157, 166, **178**, 190, *see also* self-aware proto-energy
 interaction of/with, **72**
 proto-life, 1, 2, 9, 11, 12, 24, 27, 31, **35, 36**, 46, 48, **50–53**, 54, 81, 84, 85, 88, 104, 111, 113, 120, 131, 143, 153, 171, 177, **178, 179**, 181, *see also* ℒife-precursive
 supranatural, 16–20, 61, 62, 86, 141, 178, 186
Energent proto-life, *see* Energent
 discrete & dimensional, 52
energy, 2, 5, 9, **18**, 60, 65, 157, 158, 162, 166, 181, *see also* 'energy;' proto-energy
 applied energy *E*, 8, 16, 17, 63, **65, 68**, 73, 75, 86, 114, 166
 examples, 74
 biology, 192
 negative, *see* emotive ℒife force; Intentionality
 physical, 8
'energy', *ii*, 2, 4, 5, **8**, 17, **19**, 20, **31, 50**, 54, 57, **60, 62, 63, 65–66**, 74, 78, 82, 90, 98, 100–103, **104**, 106, 107, 111, 113–115, 117, 123, 130, 131, 135, 137, 142, 148, **149**, 150, 159, **162**, 164, 165, 167, 170, 172, 179, **180**, 182, 188, 190, *see also* proto-energy
 as human essence, 80
 biological, **193**
 'density', 16, 17, **67**
 enérgeia, **19**, 47, **68–69**
 exerting, 63
 Intentionalized, 107, 122, 123, 187, 188
 of damage, 69, 103, 105, **108**
 real energy ϒ, 8, **63, 66, 68**, 74, 193
 translation, **20**, 47

energy pattern, 115, 122, **123**, 130, **131**, 132, 134, **162**, 165–168, 172, 180
energy testing, *i, vi*, 7, 40, 43, 101, **192**, 193
 validation, 35
environment, 16, 33, 72, 80, 89, 97, 131
 natural, 4, 9, 15, 16, 20, 29, 38, 45, **47**, 48, 53, 56, 59, 61, 62, 69, 73, 74, 79, 86, 91, 95, 96, 102, 106, 107, 109, 129, 135, 140–145, 149, 152, 153, 175, 186, 192
 physical, 13, 45
 'reflective', **15**, 16, 17, 20, 74, 125, 145, 157, 193, 194
 spirit, 102
 supranatural, 3, 8–12, **15–18**, 20, 24, 29, 38, 45, 47, 53, 62, 73, 85, 86, 91, 107, 129, 135, 140, 143–145, 147, 149, 152, 181, 194
 totality of, 30, 43, 145
ET, *see* energy testing
eternal, 3, 5, 8, 27, 57, 131, 132, *see also* indeterminate, infinite
 being, 3, 26, 57, 74, 90
eternity, *see* eternal
evolution, 34, 38, **43–48**, 72, 77, 88, 90, 129, 131, 183
 directed, **43–48**, 49
 undirected, **43–44**
exertion, *see* mind
existence, 3, 12, 18, 25, 29, **32**, 41, **49**, 57, **68**, 80, 81, **84**, 89, 104, **109**, 111, **137**, 138, 142, **143**, 190
 -infinite, 25
 as existentiality, 25, **33**, 81, 82, **83–86**
 as reality, 83, **84–86**
 causal regress, **27**
 mode of, 12, **28**, 29, 51
 objective, 19, 29
 physical, 7, 10, 13, 31, 105, 130, 138, 140, 147, 148, 171
 physicospirit, 23, 106, 120
 self-, 3, 41, 90
 spirit, 78, 147
experience, 6, 29, 69, 75, 76, 89, **96**, 100, 102, 109, 126, 131, 141, 154, 157, 162, 170, **173, 174**, 177, 179, 182, 186, 188, 190, 192
 as reality, 82
 conscious, 6, 18, 99, 100, 110, 112
 of mind, 6, 90
 somatic, **71**, 72, 74, 76, 78, 91, 121
 non-, **71**
 subconscious, 100, 103, 104, 106, 107, 110, 115, 117, 123

form force, *see* psyche fundamental force

Index

fundamental force, 4, 8, 39, **61**, **63**, **65**, **66**, 68, 73, 81, 113, 140, 141, 178, 190, 193, *see also* psyche fundamental force
métier force, 141

glamour, 106

habit, 83, 89, 103, 108, 135, 139, 159, 167, 180
   attributive, **78**, **79**, 102, 105, 149, 159, 163, 167, 172, 178, 186–188, *see also* Way of Being
harm, 13, 122, **124**, 132, 133, 135, **138**, 140, 151, 169, 171, **174**, 175, 177, 179, 188, 190
   -less, 89
healing, *v*, 4, 57, 62, **63**, 66, 79, 81, 82, **86**, 93, **126**, **134**, 148, 158, 160, **161**, 167, **170**, **171**, 172, 175–177, **180**, 181, 185, 191, 192, *see also* transform
   analogy to gangrene, 174, 176
   by Mina, 173, 178, **179–181**
   healer, *ii*, 79, 83, **93**, 134, 170, **171**, **172**, 190
   healing is like peeling an onion, 182
   'instant', 4, 62, 83, 109, 173
   is a whole-body experience, 172
   natural, 62, 109, **123**, 133, 151, **163**, 174, 178
   permanent, 171, **172–173**, 205
   physical, 4, 134, 139, 142, 163, 172
   psyche, **173**, 175, **178**, 179
   resistance, 95, **134**, 170, 173, 190, 205, 208, *see also* mind, subconscious
   target of, 86
health, *iii*, 24, 86, 120, 127, 129–131, 140, 164, 166, 168, 170, 180, 189, 191
   perfect, *ii*, 4, 64, 69, 79, 82, 129, **130**, 132, 163, 166, 183, 189, 193
holism, 28–30, 174, *see also* wholism
human, 5, 19, **31–32**, 41, **71**, 76, 77, 80, 84, 89, 90, 104, 109, **119**, 122, 135, 143, **161**, **169**, 191, 194
   -ize, **33**
   -ness, **31**, 41, 42, 54, **80**, 90
   first, 34, **36–37**, 52
   pairwise, *see* pairwise
   proto-, 1, 7, **60**, 88, 119, 121, **165**
      brain, 72
ʜuman, 4, 5, 7, 10, 31, 32, 34, **37**, 39, 41, 47, 52, 69, 72, **79**, 96, 99, 103, 113, 118, 119, 129, 161
humanity, 4, 14, 31, 39, 64, 88, 89, 105, 139, 144, 147, 164
   history, 6, 78, 108, 119, 121, 132, 175
   megaversal, **12**, **35**, 36, 82, 88, 135, 150

physical, 7, 12, **47**, 82, 83, 103, 105, 190
physical-born, 13, 39, 48, 76, 91, 105, 106, 144, 147, 164, 182
physicospirit, 178
spirit, 88, 190
spirit-born, 13, 39, 48, 76, 91, 106, 144, 147, 164, 182, *see also* embodiment
unembodied, **38**
universal, 12, 14, **35**, 89, 96, 106, 107, 164, 177, 182

indeterminate, 2, 3, 25, 29, 33, 50, 51, 57, 80, 84, 85, **95**, 113, 131, *see also* infinite
infinite, 2, 3, 25, 33, 50, 51, 57, 58, 83, 85, **95**, 109, 136, 155, *see also* indeterminate
   in human context, 80
   time-, 25, 27, 80
infinity, *see* infinite
injury, *vii*, 1, 69, 107, 112, 117, **122**, 126, 132, 133, 147, 154, 156, 159, 168, 174, 177, 187, 188, 191
integration, 11, **12**, 15, **24**, 32, 45, **48**, 69, 77, 91, **102**, 109, 119, 129, **130**
   example: spider-like creature, 49
   mind–body, 8, 28, 41, 44, 45, **48**, 74, 76–78, 80, **101–102**, **104**, 107, **117**, 120, 130, 131, 150, 153–155, 157, **165**, 186, 188
   full, 79
mind–body problem, 70
mind–brain, 7, **9**, 11–13, 16, 18, 40, 44, 45, 73, 75–78, 89, **99**, 101, 105, 106, 117, 120, 121, 130, 131, **142**, 144, 147, 150, 153–157, 163, 164, 181
   of proto-human, 1, 60, 72, 108, 165
intelligence, 29
   brainstem, 29
   distributed, 70
   nature of, 29
   unaware nonconscious, 27–29
Intentional machine, *see* mind
Intentionality, 1, 3, 4, 8, 9, **11**, 12, 14, 16, 19, 20, 33, 39, 44, 47, 48, **52**, 55, 61, 63, 69, 77, 78, 89, 90, 97, 98, 101–105, 108, **112**, 115, 120, **124**, 127, **130**, 132, **137**, **140**, **144**, 168, **171**, **176**, 178, **180**, **189**, 190, 192
   analogy to learning to ski, 157
   coax, **138–139**, 185
   conscious, **140**, 154
   critical moment, 50, **143**, 157, 173
   energy, 63, 120, 131, 132, **140**, **153**, **157–160**, 190
   exertion, 145, 148–150, **154**
   external, 139
   focus, 143, 148, **159**, 160
   force, 139, **141–142**, 143, **160**, **178**

Index

form, 145, 147–149
  how it works, **145–146, 148–150**
  how to exert, **151–154, 156–158**
  in the natural environment, **150–151**
  internal, 139
  of malfunction, 82
  power, **160**, 163, **169**, 170, 171, **173**, 185
  strength, 143, **160**
  subconscious, 9
  Thought, 69, 108, 120, 133, 134, **138, 143**, 153, 157, 166, 170, 171, 186, 187
    force of, **144–146**

life, 6, 13, 18, 90, 91, 164
  definition, 90
  force, 5
  is not ℒife, 80
  nonhuman, 31, 32, 34, 43, 44, 49, **66**, 67, 69, 154, *see also* nonhuman
  precursors, 47, 56
ℒife, 1, **2**, 4, 5, 7, 10–12, 24, **31**, 33, 36, 37, 39, 42, **47**, 48, **49, 52**, 53, 54, **64**, 69, 72, 79, **80**, 81, 84, 85, 87, 90, 91, **96**, 104, 105, 109, 111, 117, 119–121, 131, 133, 139, **140**, 143, 149, 150, **165**, 174, 191, 193
  -being, 99, **130**, 150
  -mind, 70, 71, 73–75
  -precursor, **2**, 11, 31, **35**, **50**, 52, 92
  force, **5**, 7, 12–14, 19, 29, 39, 56, 82, 83, 102, 104, 107, 108, 110, 126, 130, 134, 141, **149**, 152, 153, 157–159, 161, 163, 166, **171**, 175, 178, 180
    being, 7
    lightbulb analogy, 82
  force, collective, 177
  is independent of All Existence, 49
  is only ever human, **41–42**
  pairwise, *see* pairwise, *also* human ↳pairwise
  prior to, 35
ℒifeforming, 34
ℒife-precursor, **36**
  nonhuman, 194
ℒiving, 7, 10, 32, 34, 38, 42, 43, **48**, 53, 69–71, 80, 90, 131, 133, 161, 193
  body, 45
  'energy', 130, *see also* ℒiving force, 'energy'
  entity, **32**, 44, 49, 70–72, 75, 77–79, 106, 117, 119, 121, 127, 130, 141, 147, 149, 154, 160, 163, 168, 175, 193, 194
  force, 7, **14**, 19, 123, 143, 144, 148–150, 153, 154, 157, 163, 175, 193, 194

male–female, 37, 38, **39**, 47
malfunction, 82, 83, 118, 121–123, **129–132**, 140, **167, 169**, 174, 175, 180, 185, 188–190

matter, *ii*, 3–5, 8, 11, 16, 18, 20, 24, **32**, 34, 43, 45, 50, 58, **63, 65–68**, 78, 81, 83, 90, 103, **107**, 111, 120, 129, 130, **138**, **140**, 141–144, **149**, 153, 178, 191, *see also* environment ↳natural; matter–Energy
  mind over, 120
  supra-, 3, 8, 18–20, 43, **45**, **68**, 102, 107, 129, 138, 144, 147, 149, 152
matter–Energy, 5, 6, 8, 20, **63**, **66**, **67**, **69**, 71, 72, 78, 81, 83, 84, 111, 129, 130, **138**, 139–142, 155, **162**, 165, 170, 178, 191, 193, 194
  'energy' of, 79
  in relationship, 5
mbi, *see* integration ↳mind–brain
megaverse, 10, **35**, 47, 80, 90, *see also* universe
  analogies, 35
memory, 155
Mike & Molly, **39**, 44, 46–50, 52, 56, 82, 83, 85, 90, 99, 116, 137–139, 150, *see also* Twins
Mina, *i*, *v*, *vii*, 4, 10–12, 14, 16, 18, 20, 28, 29, 44, 49, 52, 55–57, 59–61, 63, 82, 101, 104, 107, 109, 112, 142, 148, 149, 162, 178, **179–181**, *see also* healing
  cited, *v*, 59, 67, 167, 168, 182, 185
  healing, 135
mind, 1, 3, 5, **6**, 7–11, 14, 19, 24, 30, 32, 38, 49, 53, **64**, **69**, 70, 79, 83, 85, 90, **96**, **100**, 102, 106, 107, 109, 110, 113, 116, **117**, 119, **130**, **132**, 135, 139, **141**, **153**, 161, 171, 191, 192, *see also* 'mind energy'
  –brain, 70
  'belief', 189
  bell of, **113–114**, **116–118**, 122, 123, 126, 167, 187, 188, 190
  conscious, *iii*, 3, 18, 75, 79, 97, **98**, **100**, 101, 108, 110, 112, 115, 120, 121, 132, 154, 157, 159, 179, 189, *see also* awareness
  -ness, **6**, 15
  analogy as water spider on pond, 109
  being, 15
  energent
    proto-life, 102
  eternal, 8
  exert, 148
  exertion, 137, 139–141, **142**, 144, 149, 151, 157, 186, 189
  human, 9, 69, 70, *see also* ℒife-, ℒife ↳mind
  indirect, 9
  is assimilative not cognitive, 76
  ℒife-, 9, 32, 70, 71, **72–75**, 77, 82, 84, 98, 99, 121, 143, 148, 150, 152–155, 157, 159, 188, *see also* mind ↳human
  manifestation of, 45

226 Index

nonhuman, 5, **70–72**
physical, 72, 73, 76
physically instantiated, 10, 18, **72–73**, 75–78, 89, 130, 150, **151**, **153**, 155–157, 159, 181, 194
self-actualize, 83, **97**, 112, 113, 118, 122, 129, 147, 152, 167
spirit, 73, 76, 152
subconscious, *iii*, 3, 13, 14, 19, 53, 57, 63, 64, 75, 77, 78, 83, 88, 97, **98–102**, 103–106, 109, 110, 112, **115**, 116, 117, **118**, **119**, 120, 121, 124, **132**, 133, 134, 136, 140, **151**, **154**, 155, 157–159, 163, 167, 172, 173, 179, 186, 188, 189, *see also* awareness
amalgamation, **78**, 130
an Intentional machine, 83, 90, 102, 117, **118**, 133, 154, 159, 165–167, **169**, 172
analogy as paper, 105
awareness, *see* awareness
'belief', 102, **103**, 106–108, **117**, **118**, 122, **125**, 126, 127, 130–133, 164–166, **167**, 168, **169**, 170–172, 185, 186, 188, 191
'energy of', 102
letting go, 126
reconciliation, 100, 111, 180
resistance, 95, 112, **134**, 170, 190, 205, *see also* healing
self-actualize, 176
subconscious–conscious, 21, 78, 89, 97, **99**, **101**, **102**, 111–113, 115, **117**, 122, 126, **130–131**, 132, 146, 147, 166, **169**, 170, 171, 174, 177, 178, 180, 182, 183, 185, 187, 189
un-, **30–31**
wholistic, 98, 102, 111, **118**, 119, 154, 179
'mind energy', 3, **104**, 108, 134, 138, 139, 142, 144, 146, **153**, **154**, 156, 158, 159, 173
mind–body, *see* integration
mindset, *ii*, 7–9, 12–14, 38, 77, 88, 117, 121, 123, **125**, 126, **130**, 132–134, 144, **147**, 148, 149, **162**, 164–167, 174, 175, 187–189, 191
addiction, 12, 13, 170, 174, 177, 180
collective, 89, 126, 132, **134**, 147, 164, 167, 170
type-, 38
mitosis, *see also* emergent ↳ birth

NCC, *see* Negative Collective Consciousness
negate, 90, 95, 106, 130, 134, 148, 151, 161, 166, 167, 170–172, 188, 190, *see also* neutralize
Negative Collective Consciousness, **13**, 88, 89, 96, 101, **104**, 164, **170**, 171, 175, 177, **179**, 182
local, 175, 182
neutralize, 14, 114, 116, 124, **148**, 150, 160, 163, 174, 175, 178, **179**, 180, 182, 190, 191, *see also* negate
nonautonomy, *see* autonomy
nonhuman, 5, 29, 70, 72, 76, 77, 80, 90, 117, 130, 132, 133, 135, 194, *see also* animal, life

omniexistence, 83, 84, 159, 189
omnipotence, 83, **84**, 135, 159, 166, 189
omnipresence, 83, **84**, 135, 159, 189
omniscience, 83, **84**, 110, 159, 189
own-self, **5**, 6, 30, 75, 77, 89, 100, 102, 104, 109, 114, 137, 138, 152, 191

pain, *i*, *iii*, *v*, *vii*, 74, 102, 106, 120, 124, 133, 158, 171, 173, 174, **175**, 176, 177, **179**, 180, 181, **182**, 186
healing is like peeling an onion, 173, 177
pairwise, 1, 2, **38**, **39**, 40, 52, 53, 67, 90, 183
human, 37, 49, 143
kinship, **36**, 39, 52
permission, 45, 134, 185, **186**, 210
person, 4, 29, 42, 78–80, 82, 85, 88, 91, 96, 109, 110, 119, 122, 123, **130**, **135**, **141**, 170, 174, 179
-ness, **4**, **31–32**, **41–42**, 50, 76, 90
emergent, 6, 48
physical, 18, 106, 125, 133, 142, 147, 150, 151, 153, 185, 186, 189, 193, 194
physicospirit, 21, 193
spirit, 6–9, 16–18, 20, 44, 49, 56, 106, 132, 142, 145, 147, 148, 171, 185, 186, 190, 193, **194**
person, **1**, 3, 5, 7, 12, **32**, 33, **37**, 41, 49, 52, 69, 72, 78, 79, 96, 104, 111, 113, 129, **141**, 143, **152**, 161, 178
spirit, 146
personness, **79**
Philosophy with a capital-P, **15**, 29, 35, 37, 40–42, 64, 65, 70, 77, 78, 80, 83, 85, 88, 90, 120, 127, 130, 154
physical, 6, 8, 12, 15, 16, 19, 51, 167, *see also* natural; environment
birth, 6
entity, 17, 18, 74
non-, 15, 17, 69, 73, 90
parents, 6
physicospirit, 1, **7**, 9, 12, 13, 15, 44–46, **48**, 53, 56, 76, 78, 95, 106, 117, **152**
embodiment, *see* embodiment
life, 7
picosecond, **4**, 14, 55, 109, 142, 150, **157**
proto-energy, 45, 60, 97

Index

proto-human
  Neanderthal, 1
proto-life, *see* Energent
proto-love, **39–40**, 52, 177
  LOVE, 40
  love, 40
psyche, *i*, 15, 24, 49, **64**, **79–81**, 90, 96, 97, 101, **117**, **170**, 174, 175, 177, 181, *see also* consciousness
  healing, **173**
  time and space infinite, 83
psyche fundamental force, **140–143**, 149, 178
  form force, 141, 142
  switch force, 141, 142
psyche healing, **190**

quantum entanglement, 27, 53, 61, 62
quinta essentia, **28**

real energy ϒ, *see* 'energy'
Reality, 80
reality, 5, 8, 11, 18, 24, **28**, 29, 30, **33**, 48, **51**, 64, 82, 83, **84–86**, 89, 91, 95, **98**, 100, **102**, 103, 105, **107**, **109**, 111, 120, 144, 149, 162, 165, 166, 171, 174, 176, 177
  arising in consciousness, 80
  biological, 132, 147, 150
  causative, 25
  chosen, 38
  Energent proto-life, **52**
  experience, 82
  fundamental, 31, 37
  human, 34, 131, 144, 168, 178, 185, 192
  Intentional, 45, 125, 126
  natural, 40, 103
  objective, 5, 6, 71
  physical, 8, 58, 66, 123, 148, 164, 168, 185, 186, **190–192**
  physicospirit, 7, 13, 78, 79, 96, 98, 105, 106, 120, 130, 136, 147
  spirit, 12, 14, 140, 168
  subjective, 5, 6, 71, 105
  supranatural, 40, 47
Reconciliation, 14, 101, 106, 182
redolent with impression, 75, 115, 121

sapience, 30
sapient, 28, 47, 58
science, *i*, *vi*, 4, 28, 29, 34, 40, 43, 50, 58–60, 62, 65–67, 70, 77, 90, 96, 127, 141, 142, 144, 155, 156, 159, 163, 165, 191, 192
self, 145, 174, *see also* own-self
  emergent, *see* emergent ⌊self
  ⌊Life-, 19, 77, 97, 150, 151, **152**, 153, 175, 178, 179
  physical, 6, 9, 10, 74, 75, 150, 151, 154

spirit, 9, 10, 12, 73, 89, 127, 150–153, 181, 186, 187, 193
self-actualize
  mind, *see* mind
self-aware, *see* aware
self-aware proto-energy, 2, 4, 9, 43, 85, **96**, 104, 110, 120, 129, 131, **152**, 165, 166
  being, **2**, 4, 12, 24, 82, 85, 86, 91, 111, 113, 123, 133, 164
  person, 1, **6**, 12, 14, 15, **32**, 80, 82, 102
  self, 3, 33, 45, 48, 51, **99**, 102–105, 107, 113, 115, 116, 122, 126, **130**, 131, **152**, **153**, 167, 174, **177**, 182, 188
self-awareness, 5, 6, 12, 31, 32, 41, **49**, 50, 52, **64**, 71, 75, **76–77**, 80, **97**, 115, 174, 177, *see also* awareness
  faux, 71
  first instance, **36**
  human, 5, 6
  non-, 32
  nonhuman, 5, 6, 71
self-physical, 73
sentient, 28, 30, 47, 58
sex, 2, 3, 8, **37–39**, 53
SOA, *see* awareness ⌊state(s) of
SOB, *see* being ⌊state(s) of
space, 3, 33, 34, 50, 52, 54, **57–59**, 62, 65, 68, **80**, **84**, 85, 113, 137, 140, 144, 153, *see* universe
spirit, *see* awareness; embodiment; environment; existence; humanity; person, reality; self
spirit attack, 132, 148, 149, 159, 185, 186, 189, 190
  direct, **186**
  indirect, **186–189**
spirit-aware, *see* awareness
subconscious, 192, *see* mind
suffering, *iii*, *v*, 13, 40, 106, 164, 171, 173, 175–178, 181, **182**, 189
supramatter, *see* matter; *see also* environment ⌊supranatural
supranatural, *see* Energent; environment; matter; reality; world
switch force, *see* psyche fundamental force

tedious, 3, **46**, 142, 144
thinking–feeling, **6**, 8, 32, 41, 75, 77, 98, **100**, 101, 109–111, 115, 120, 141, 146, 147, 154, 193, 194, *see also* awareness–experiential; Thought
thought, 138–141, 146, 158, 165, 173, 193
Thought, **6**, 8, 14, 32, 45, 48, 57, 63, 75, 77, 98, **100**, 103, 104, 110, 111, 115, 116, 120, 123, 133, **137**, 138, 140, 141, 143, 146, 147, 153, 154, 159, **162**, 170, 171,

173, **179**, 180, 187, 190, 191, *see also* Intentionality
conscious, 19, 108, 110–112, 115, 122, 127, 155, 159, 173, 177, 183, 185
force, 140, 160, 173, **178**
force of, 148, 149, 153
structure, 179, 180
sub-, **110**, 111, 136, 154, 156
subconscious, 108, 185
time, 2, 3, 33, 34, 50, 52, 54, 57, 62, 65, 68, 80, **81**, **84**, 85, 113, 131, 137, 153, 191
timekeeping, 81
examples, 81
transcend, **10**, 12, 24, 27–29, 71, 76
transcendent, 33
transform, 4, 82, **86**, 109, 148, 158, 160, **161**, 163, 165, 167, 170, 172, 173, *see also* healing
translate, **41**, **62**
transliterate, 99, 101, 121, 153, 155, *see* brain
trauma, 100, 106, 122, 154, 169, 173, 176, 180
Twins, **36–39**, 45, 47, 49, *see also* Mike & Molly

Ultraculture, *see* culture
unembodiment, *see* embodiment
UNI, *see* unaware nonconscious intelligence *in* awareness; intelligence
universe, *i*, 2, 6, 9–15, 18–20, 25, 28, 31–33, 38, 50, 53, 55–58, **59**, **65**, **67**, 69, 73, 81, 82, 88, 91, 103, 104, 106, 107, 109, 112, 123, 131, 133–135, 137, 141, 142, **144**, 149, 170, 179, 182, 188, 190, 193, *see also* megaverse
Big Bang, 25, 48, 61
builder, 45, 52, 54, 97, 135, 143, 149, 178, 180
designed for life, 29
megaverse, 135
natural (physical), 8, 20, 96, 140
original Way of Being, 28, *see also* Way of Being
Primoverse, 44, 47–49, 56, 138, 150
prior to, 35
space, 2
unmind, *see* mind

WOB, *see* Way of Being

Way of Being, 2, 3, **4**, 5, 9, 11, 12, 18–20, 26, 28, **30–31**, 34, 35, 37, 39, 43, 44, 52, 59, 60, 76, 78, **80**, 82–84, **86–88**, 89, 90, 99, 100, **104**, 105, 111, 116, 122, 131, **132**, 135, 138, 142, 144, **145**, 148, 149, 153, 168
Human, 164
All Existence, 11, **26**, 34, **60**, 67, 80, 82, 86
as Way of Being, **26**, 91, 161
attributive, **5**, **78**, **79**, 89, 101, 108, 114, 120, 122, 123, **130**, 131, 132, 134, 136, 149, 159, 163, **164–167**, 168, **169**, 170, 171, 174, 188, 189, *see also* habit
emergent, *ii, vii*, 3–5, 10, 13, 67, 69, 78, 83, 84, 86, 101, 102, 104, 106, 107, 109, 113, 114, 116, 117, 120, 123, 124, 126, 129–131, **132**, **133**, 134, 135, 142, 145, 152, 158, **162–164**, 165, 167, 170, 172, 174, 189
'energy' of, 78, 79, 86, 130, 133, 167, 171, 188, 191
Human, 10, 38, 45, 49, 52, 54, 88, 89, 97, 107, 116, 131, 171, **179**, 181, 182, 186
human-Intentionalized, 34, 47, 67, 104, 111
individual, 38, 88, 89, 162, 171
nonconscious, 26
original, 28, 129, **133**
own-self, 30
physical body, 89, 163, **188**, 189
self-organized, **87–88**
computer metaphor, 87
subconscious, 79, 108
type, 38
wellbeing, *ii, iii*, 79, 120, **124**, 129, 130, 164, 166, 168, 189
own-self, 5
physical, 25
wholism, **28**, 29–31, **32**, 34, 39, 41, 43, 44, 77, 78, 97–99, 102, 110, 111, 120, 145, 154, 162, 172, 176, 177, *see also* holism
world (physical or spirit), *see* environment ⌊natural or ⌊supranatural

you are not a victim, 92, 109, 131, 164, 188, 199
you are not your body, 3, 12, 23, 24, 31, 84, 91

zygote, 54, 55

www.ingramcontent.com/pod-product-compliance
Lightning Source LLC
Chambersburg PA
CBHW020457030426
42337CB00011B/134